Eye Was There

Eye Was There

A Patient's Guide to Coping
with the Loss of an Eye

Charles B. Slonim, M.D.
Amy Z. Martino, M.D.

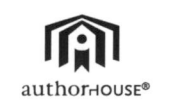

authorHOUSE®

AuthorHouse™
1663 Liberty Drive
Bloomington, IN 47403
www.authorhouse.com
Phone: 1-800-839-8640

First published by AuthorHouse 07/13/2011

ISBN: 978-1-4567-6663-4 (sc)
ISBN: 978-1-4567-6661-0 (ebk)

Library of Congress Control Number: 2011907070

Printed in the United States of America

Dedication

To the three wonderful women in my life: Barrie, Arlie and Emma

In memory of my grandfather, Adolf Mueller

Acknowledgement

I am extremely grateful for the significant contributions to this book from my student, Amy Z. Martino, M.D.

I would like to thank Porex Surgical, Inc. and Integrated Orbital Implants, Inc. for allowing me to use some of their schematic illustrations and images for this book.

Contents

Introduction

The most treasured of the five basic human senses is sight. The ability to see provides an individual a considerable amount of independence whether or not other physical disabilities exist. Looking at familiar faces of friends and family, gazing at a scenic landscape, staring into a mirror at one's reflection, glancing across a room as someone enters it, or peeking into a box of candy impart a sense of freedom to a person who would otherwise require a description of the view from a sighted person.

The complete loss of sight can be devastating; however, the loss of a single eye can be equally as disturbing. Patients who are told that the removal of their diseased or blind and painful eye is "only a matter of time" have very few sources of information, outside their doctor's office, from which they can learn about what to expect both before and after the surgery. Unfortunately, the doctor or the doctor's staff might not have the time or may not be equipped to handle the variety of questions that patients commonly ask. Also, many of the questions arise after the patient has left the doctor's office.

This book is intended for people who have recently experienced the loss of an eye or are considering the removal of an eye. It is also intended for their caretakers, their family members, and their friends. It is meant as a source of information as to their available preoperative, surgical, and postoperative options. It is a basic manual to explain the different surgical options available to the patient awaiting surgery. It is a source of historical and current information regarding the manufacturing, care, and handling of artificial eyes and orbital prostheses that are worn after surgery.

Anatomy

An understanding of the basic anatomy of the orbit and the eye is necessary to appreciate the relationships between the parts of the eye and orbit that are surgically removed and the parts that are left behind and eventually support the artificial eye (i.e., the prosthesis). For the purpose of this chapter, the eye socket will be divided into two sections: the orbit and the eye.

Anatomy of the Orbit

The orbit is a recessed bony cavity in the face positioned on either side of the nose. Each orbit contains a number of soft tissues and structures including the eyeball, muscles, nerves, blood vessels, fat, and fascia. Each orbit is shaped like a pear, with the top of the pear pointing toward the back of the head. Each orbit has four main inside surfaces or walls, which are described by their relative position in each orbit. There is a "roof" on the top and a "floor" on the bottom of each orbit. There is a medial wall (closest to the nose) and a lateral wall (closest to the ear). There are a total of seven different bones that make up each orbit. Some of the bones have holes in them to allow the passage of nerves and blood vessels. The opening edge of the orbit crates a round shape and is called the orbital rim.

The orbit also contains six extraocular muscles that are attached to the outside surface of the eyeball called the sclera (the white part of the eye). These muscles are responsible for eye movements. The eyeball is actually positioned in the center of these muscles. The optic nerve extends from the back of the eyeball through the center of the muscles;

it continues through the back of the orbit and goes through a hole in the back of the orbit and connects with the brain. Surrounding the extraocular muscles, the optic nerve, and the eyeball is the orbital fat, which helps to support and cushion the eye in the orbit. The lacrimal gland, which produces watery tears, is positioned in the upper and outer portion of each orbit. The lacrimal drainage system, which helps drain the tears away from the eye, is located in the lower and inner portion of each orbit. Positioned in front of the orbital rims are the eyelids.

Anatomy of the Eye

The eye is a very complex organ that is made up of many parts. Each part has a specific function, and together these parts are responsible for creating a visual image which is interpreted as vision.

There are three main layers of the eyeball. The outer layer is a protective layer made of a very tough, fibrous tissue. In the front of the eye this tissue is a clear dome, called the cornea, and it represents about 20 percent of the entire surface of the outer layer. A healthy cornea has no blood vessels in it; it is the only part of the eye that can be transplanted. When a cornea becomes cloudy due to disease or trauma, a surgeon can replace the central portion of the damaged cornea with a clear cornea that has been donated from a deceased organ donor; this is called a corneal transplant. The other 80 percent of the outer layer is white and is called the sclera. Attached to the sclera are the six extraocular muscles, which are responsible for all of the eye movements.

The middle layer of the eye contains extremely delicate structures that include the iris, ciliary body, and choroid. The iris is the colored portion of the eye that gives someone the appearance of having blue, green or brown eyes. In the center of the iris is the pupil which is the black circular hole that allows the light to go through to the back of the eye. The pupil regulates the amount of light that goes into the eye. The pupil opens widely in dark light and closes to a small hole in bright light.

The ciliary body produces the fluid (aqueous) that fills the eye and maintains a certain pressure needed to keep the eye in a round shape. Inside the front of the eye is an area between the back of the cornea and the front of the iris; this area is called the filtration angle, where the aqueous eventually drains from the eye. The production of aqueous from the ciliary body and the drainage of aqueous from the filtration angle must be kept in a constant balance so that the pressure inside the eye remains fairly constant. If the drainage system becomes defective, then the pressure in the eye will go up. The condition where the pressure in the eye is too high is called glaucoma. If the pressure in the eye remains too high for too long, then damage will occur to the optic nerve. Damage to the optic nerve initially causes peripheral (side) vision loss, which can eventually lead to central vision loss and blindness. The optic nerve has approximately 1.6 million nerve fibers that go to the brain. Modern surgical techniques have not been developed yet to repair a damaged optic nerve; it is mainly for this reason that total eye transplants are not yet possible.

Behind the ciliary body is the choroid, which is made of many blood vessels. The choroid is sandwiched between the sclera of the outer layer and the retina of the inner layer. The choroid brings nourishment to both of these layers. Behind the iris and pupil lies the clear crystalline lens of the eye. Like the lens of a camera, the natural crystalline lens of the eye is responsible for receiving the light that enters the eye and focusing that light onto the retina in the back of the eye. Over time, the crystalline lens can become cloudy or opaque. When this occurs, the cloudy lens is referred to as a cataract.

The retina is a transparent tissue that lines the surface of the back of the eye and is in front of the choroid. The retina contains the photoreceptor cells known as the rods and cones. Photoreceptor cells receive the light which has been focused by the lens and changes the light into an electrical impulse. This electrical impulse is then transmitted through the optic nerve to the occipital lobe of the brain, where it is translated into a visual image.

There are two fluids inside the eye: the aqueous fluid and the vitreous gel. The aqueous fluid fills the anterior chamber, which is the space between the iris and the cornea. The vitreous gel fills the space inside the back of the eye behind the lens and in front of the retina

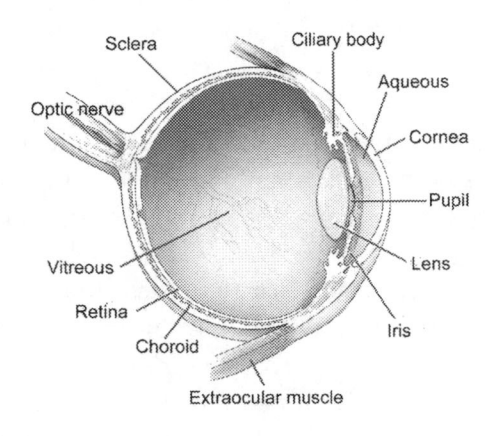

Epidemiology

The number of surgeries to remove an eye for medical reasons has declined over time due to earlier detection of diseases and more conservative management. The choice of surgical procedure to remove an eye has also changed over time. Initially, doctors were performing mostly enucleations, in which the entire eyeball and some of the nerve that connected it to the brain were removed. However, over the last few decades, many doctors are shifting to an alternative surgery called an evisceration, which involves removing just the inner contents of the eyeball.[1] This way, the outer shell of the eye (the sclera) remains with all of its muscles attached, so that it may look and move more like the other eye.

Losing an eye does not discriminate based on age, gender, socioeconomic status, or lifestyle. However, young males of lower socioeconomic status experience ocular trauma and subsequent loss of an eye more than any other group. The number of eyes removed in each country around the world varies annually just as much as the reasons for removing them. Here in the United States, trauma is the most common event that results in the loss of an eye. The U.S. National Center for Health Statistics' Health Interview Survey estimates that around 2.4 million eye injuries occur in the U.S. each year.[2] Another study has shown that approximately 3 people out of every 100,000 suffer a penetrating eye injury every year.[3] As a result of these eye injuries, 50,000 people permanently lose part or all of their vision. Ninety percent of all eye injuries can be prevented by using protective eyewear.[4] In a study involving 2,276 patients who were hospitalized as a result of eye injuries, 2,416 eyes were injured (140 patients injured both eyes). Forty-seven percent (1,070 patients) were children, who often sustained the most severe injuries. The male-to-female ratio was 4.3 to 1. Most patients retained good vision, 3.7 percent (89 eyes) lost vision totally, and 2 percent (48 eyes) had to be removed.[5] According to the Society for the Prevention of Blindness, between 10,000 and 12,000 people per year lose an eye. Approximately 50 percent or more of these eyes are lost due to an accident.[6]

Whether due to a motor vehicle accident, assault during an altercation, work-related injury, or even gunshot wound, patients who lose an eye due to trauma tend to be young males under age thirty. Work-related injuries often result from hammering nails; either the entire nail flies up and punctures the eye, or a piece of metal breaks off of the nail and hits the eye. Eye injury is a significant health problem in the United States, second only to cataract as a cause of visual impairment.

If the eyeball is punctured or deflated from the trauma, it is termed an open-globe (see: Surgery: Timing: Open globe injury). Around two hundred thousand open-globe injuries occur worldwide each year.[6] Other common reasons for removing an eye in adults not related to trauma include cancer of the eye, especially melanoma; severe infection inside the eye, called endophthalmitis; and a blind eye that later becomes too painful to manage with medication or surgery. In children, many devastating eye injuries are due to preventable causes such as BB guns, paintball guns, and ice hockey.

Many of the eyes removed from children that are not due to accidents are the result of a cancer called retinoblastoma. Pediatricians examine the eyes of all newborns at birth and at every subsequent checkup after that to detect this uncommon, although devastating, childhood cancer of the eye as early as possible. If the cancer is detected early enough, medications may be used for treatment; this is referred to as chemotherapy. However if the retinoblastoma tumor is advanced, surgery to remove the eye is often the best form of treatment to prevent it from spreading to other parts of the body.

Worldwide, especially in third-world countries, serious eye conditions that result in the removal of an eye include infections and tumors. Delayed diagnosis and treatment, as well as little or no access to eye care specialists, likely explain much of this phenomenon. Although the number of enucleations may parallel that in the United States, there are more exenterations performed abroad. An exenteration involves removing the entire eyeball plus some of the surrounding tissues (such as muscle, fat, and possibly bone). For example, those living in a tropical climate in underdeveloped countries have a higher incidence of squamous cell carcinoma, a cancer that begins on the eyelids or surface of the eye and that can spread to surrounding bone. By the time that person seeks medical attention, the cancer may have spread very widely inside the orbit. The only option for treatment and a possible cure with widespread orbital tumors is an exenteration.

Causes

There are a variety of reasons (e.g., medical and surgical indications) that may prompt a surgeon to suggest that an eye may need to be removed. A number of factors must be taken into consideration before proceeding with surgery. These factors include the level of vision, the level of pain and discomfort, the risk to the good eye, the risk to the patient's general health in the case of a malignant tumor, the physical appearance of the eye, and the quality of life.

Probably the most important considered factor is the level of vision that exists in the eye in question. Visual acuity is the measure of the ability of the eye to see certain images of different sizes and shapes at different distances. Typically, this is determined by having a patient read an eye chart with multiple lines of letters or numbers that get progressively smaller as one reads further down the chart. The written or documented notation of a visual acuity is indicated in the form of a fraction (e.g., 20/40), which refers to distances measured in feet. This fraction is referred to as a Snellen notation of vision named after the Dutch ophthalmologist, Herman Snellen, who developed the chart in 1862.

The numerator (top number) indicates at what distance the patient must stand from the chart in order to be able to see a certain sized letter, number or shape. The standard distance for viewing the eye chart in the eye doctor's office is calibrated (mirrored) to a twenty-foot length. Therefore the numerator is usually indicated as 20. This means that the patient was able to see the identified letter at 20 feet. Outside the United States where the metric system of measurements is used, this is calibrated to 6 meters, which equals 19.69 feet. Therefore a visual acuity metric notation of 6/12 would be equivalent to 20/40. The denominator (the bottom number) is the distance that a population of persons with normal vision could see the same-sized letter on the same line of the eye chart. For example, suppose a patient can only see down to the 20/40 line on the eye chart. The size of letter or image that this patient can see at twenty feet can be seen by persons with normal vision at forty feet away, or twice the distance.

The definition of legal blindness differs around the world. In the United States, the definition of legal blindness is defined as a visual acuity in the better eye with the best possible prescribed glasses of 20/200 (the biggest "E" on the chart) or worse, or the peripheral field of vision (side vision) restricted to twenty degrees or less in the better eye (tunnel vision).

When the letters on the eye chart can no longer be seen because of poor or deteriorating vision, then the eye doctors refers to a different nonnumerical (i.e., non-Snellen) system of indicating a visual acuity (e.g., NLP, LP, HM, CF). Being able to count fingers held in front of the patient within a few feet of their eye is referred to as count fingers (CF) vision at, for example, two feet. If the patient cannot delineate the number of fingers held up by the eye doctor, they will be asked if they can see hand movement. The doctor will wave his or her hand in front of the patient's face. If the patient can see the movement of the hand, this is referred to as hand motions (HM) vision. If hand motions are not visible to the patient, the eye doctor will ask the patient if they can see a bright light source shined into their eye. If the light is visible, this is referred to as light perception (LP) vision. If the patient can tell from which direction the point source of light is coming from, then this is referred to a "light perception with projection" vision. If no light perception is seen by the patient to the brightest available beam of light, then this is referred to as no light perception (NLP) vision. A no light perception eye is considered to be a totally blind eye. It is at the NLP level of vision that an ophthalmologist will consider removing an eye depending on the circumstances surrounding the medical necessity to remove that eye.

Birth Defects

There are occasions when infants are born with birth defects that directly affect the eye. Three such conditions are microphthalmos, congenital cystic eye, and rarely, anophthalmos. Microphthalmos is a condition where the eye is extremely small and blind. A rare condition called congenital anophthalmos is where the infant is born without an eye in the socket. The term "socket" refers to the space contained within the orbital bones that contains the eyeball. The socket surrounds and protects the eye.

When conditions like these are encountered, the surgeon's attention is directed to the growth of the orbital bones surrounding the eyeball. Without a normal sized eye growing within the bony socket, the bones of the socket may not grow normally to an adult size. This can cause a facial asymmetry as the bony orbit that surrounds the good eye grows to a normal size. Reconstructive surgery of the socket usually involves the removal of the defective eye and replacing it with progressively enlarging orbital implants or socket expanders. These devices, simply by their presence in the socket, can stimulate the bones of the orbit to grow simultaneously with the other normal socket. The goal is to create facial symmetry as the infant grows through childhood and into adolescence, at which time further growth of the socket stops.

Blind and Painful

The most common medical justifications for removing an eye is when that eye is blind (i.e., NLP) *and* painful. Regardless of the cause of the blindness, a chronically painful eye can produce significant morbidity to the patient. The pain can be due to a variety of causes. It can be the result of direct irritation or inflammation of nerve fibers. It can be the result of uncontrolled high pressure in the eye (i.e., glaucoma). Ironically, eye pain is also associated with an eye that has lost the ability to maintain its pressure inside or has no inside pressure. This is referred to as a phthisical eye. Comparing a normal eye with pressure to a phthisical eye with no pressure is like comparing a grape to a raisin. An eye with no internal pressure shrinks into a small, collapsed, irregular shape. An eye with no pressure can hurt just as bad as an eye with too much pressure.

Eye pain of any sort can make a patient irritable, cranky, uncomfortable, unpleasant, and depressed. Some patients require prescription pain medications in order to relieve the eye pain. These pain medications can have a negative effect on the general well-being of the patient and frequently will not completely alleviate all of the eye pain. As with any narcotic painkiller medication that is taken chronically, drug dependency can occur.

In the vast majority of cases, when the blind and painful eye is removed, so is the pain associated with it. Removing the eye frequently allows patients to get on with their life, which has been temporarily interrupted by the eye pain.

Painful and Unsightly but Not Totally Blind

On occasion, an eye might be painful and unsightly but not totally blind. This is a major challenge for both the surgeon and the patient. On one hand, any vision, even light perception vision, is better than no vision at all. If something happened to the good eye, then at least the person could see when lights are turned on and off. On the other hand, an eye with chronic pain affects a person's quality of life. Sometimes sacrificing a light-perception or hand-motion eye with absolutely no chance of improvement or rehabilitation allows the person to move on with his or her life. The removal of this kind of painful or unsightly but not totally blind eye greatly improves the future quality of the person's life and the lives of close friends and family.

These patients require long discussions with their surgeons before considering a surgery to remove the eye. Some surgeons will not remove an eye under these circumstances. Many surgeons will send these patients for second and third opinions prior to any surgery. The length of time that the eye has been painful will have a lot to do with the decision process. Occasionally, a painful eye may become more tolerable over time.

Trauma

The most common cause of a sudden loss of vision is trauma. Eye injury is a leading cause of monocular blindness in the United States.[7] This includes direct trauma (e.g., high-speed projectiles, foreign bodies) and indirect trauma (e.g., blunt object to the orbit).

The eye is an easy target when left unprotected during contact sports or racquet sports, where a projectile is propelled at high velocities. Many of these traumatic injuries can result in hemorrhages or bleeding in the eye, or actually lacerate the eyeball, which is referred to as an open globe injury. Open globe injuries frequently result in a loss of some of the internal tissues and/or structures from inside the eye (see: Surgery: Timing: Open globe injury). With the loss of these structures or as a result of a severe hemorrhage in the eye, the eye may eventually lose light perception and become blind. Protective eye wear can prevent the majority of traumatic eye injuries.

Intraocular Tumors

Malignant tumors or cancers can originate inside the eye. These tumors can develop at birth (e.g., retinoblastoma) or later in life (e.g., choroidal melanoma). The capability of such tumors to spread to other parts of the body depends on the type of tumor. The diagnosis of an intraocular tumor can be difficult. Most tumors found elsewhere in the body can be biopsied. A biopsy is where a small piece of the tumor is surgically removed and sent to a pathologist to determine its tissue type and its degree of malignancy, or tendency to spread and eventually cause death. Unfortunately, tumors inside the eye are rarely biopsied because the biopsy procedure itself can cause significant damage to the eye.

With most tumors, removing the eye with the tumor intact usually allows the patient the best chance of a cure and a high survival rate. Of course, survival rates are dependent on the length of time that the tumor existed, the degree of malignancy of the tumor, and the complete removal of tumor. Occasionally, further treatment (e.g., chemotherapy or radiation therapy) may be required even after the eye and the tumor have been removed.

Cosmetic

Sometimes blind eyes become unsightly and cosmetically unattractive. This can be the result of a birth defect of the eye. This can also be a result from the original trauma that may have blinded the eye. Phthisical eyes typically have cloudy or opaque corneas and collapsed scleras, and they are frequently red all the time. A cosmetically unattractive eye can occur from having multiple surgeries to repair an eye. An unsightly eye tends to draw the attention of other people; person-to-person conversations usually begin with eye to eye contact. Tinted glasses can frequently mask or camouflage an unattractive eye, but they also reduce the visibility of the good eye. A patch can also be worn, but many people feel that a patch draws more attention to them than the unsightly eye itself.

In cases where a blind eye is unsightly and a scleral shell and/or cosmetic contact lens (see: Cosmesis without Surgery) were not successful in restoring the appearance of the original eye, the removal of the eye may be an option.

Psychology of Organ Loss

Losing an eye can be devastating, both emotionally and physically. Whether the surgery to remove an eye was done on an emergency basis or was preplanned and performed on an elective basis, no one is ever prepared to lose an eye. A process of grieving is necessary to lead to the eventual acceptance of losing a part of the body. However, the extremes of avoiding grief altogether and excessive preoccupation with the loss can also create psychological disturbances.

As with any significant loss, such as the loss of a loved one, patients who have an eye removed often go through five predictable stages of grieving: denial, anger, bargaining, grief, and acceptance. Not everyone passes through these in order, but eventually the goal is for all grieving persons to reach acceptance. Eye doctors may only observe their patients as they experience the initial denial phase and seem to be handling life with only one eye very well. Patients may be reluctant to express feelings of anger to their doctor—whether the anger is directed toward the person who may have caused the injury or even at the doctor for not being able to "save the eye." The bargaining phase occurs as people may try to negotiate with their supreme being (God) to restore sight in the lost eye or help create an eye transplant that would restore sight, in exchange for promising to, for example, better control their blood sugar from diabetes. The grief stage is where people begin to realize that their life is forever changed, and they may experience deep sadness and anguish. This stage can often mimic or lead to depression. Patients should be closely monitored to watch for signs of suicidal or even homicidal thoughts. Referral to a mental health professional is imperative in these cases.

Most people experience two types of grief following the loss of an eye: loss of body image and loss of function.[8] Loss of body image refers to the emotions that people experience in reaction to the way others perceive them. Some people may feel embarrassed, ashamed, or anxious around family members and friends. These emotions are strongest in the weeks immediately following surgery—for example, the time when an artificial eye cannot yet be fitted because postoperative healing continues. Even with a well-made ocular prosthesis in place with a wide range of movement, some people may have a sense of being different and a fear of strangers staring and finding out that their eye is not real.

When greeting someone face to face, someone with one eye may avoid making eye contact and therefore may fear that he or she is being perceived as vulnerable and submissive. Rarely, the grief may lead to depression, anxiety, and sexual problems. In these cases, one should seek the guidance of a professional psychologist or psychiatrist in order to deal with these kinds of problems. After a prosthesis is put in place, around 90 percent of patients are satisfied with the way they look. In fact, 80 percent of those patients say others cannot even tell that they have only one eye.[9]

The final stage is acceptance. People are then at peace with living a monocular life. They realize that they can return to doing and seeing almost everything they were able to before they lost an eye.

Loss of function refers to an alteration in sensation. Certainly with the loss of one eye, a person will notice some changes in their visual perception. Some describe noticeable changes in their side vision and their depth perception. Typically, over time the brain and body adapt to being monocular.

People may bump into objects while walking as they learn new cues for depth. Extended head movements to the side of the lost eye will help compensate for the reduced peripheral vision to that side. Eventually the brain will develop a two-dimensional depth perception by watching the changes in object size or by observing the positional changes of an object as one approaches or moves away from the object. These maneuvers will help compensate for a reduction in depth perception. Others may reach for something multiple times before finally grasping it. Placing an object, such as a glass, on the edge of a table may be more difficult than it appears when there is a loss of depth perception.

Driving can be especially tricky. In all states, driving with one eye is legal. Most states require that one eye has a visual acuity equal to or better than 20/40 and must have a normal peripheral field of vision. Each person should check with their state's Department of Motor Vehicles to verify the laws and regulations. Even though a person meets their state requirements and may be legal to drive, precautions should be taken to make sure that person feels safe enough driving on the road. Many people need extra time to learn how to compensate for a loss of depth perception when they lose an eye. A simple extended turn of their head to the left or right can significantly increase their field of vision. They may also need to relearn how to judge the distance of a car in front of them, or when to start slowing down for a traffic light or traffic sign. Some state laws may require that one-eyed persons repeat driving tests more frequently to ensure that the visual acuity in the remaining eye is strong enough and continues to meet driving criteria. After becoming acclimated to having one eye, the vast majority of people typically return to all of their previously enjoyed activities without even realizing they have a prosthesis.

People with severely decreased or absent vision, whether in one or both eyes, can experience something called Charles-Bonnet syndrome. In this syndrome, vivid, complex visual hallucinations are seen, even though the person is mentally sound. Many are embarrassed to tell others about what they are seeing for fear they will be called insane. These are strictly visual hallucinations; no other sensory hallucinations such as hearing, tasting, or smelling things are present. People can perceive a wide variety of shapes, faces, animals, flowers, or even cartoon characters. The hallucinations are believed to be the brain making up images because the eye is no longer providing them. Treatment is rarely necessary; the hallucinations typically last for a year or two before disappearing as suddenly as they began.[10]

Cosmesis without Surgery

When a blind eye is not painful but unattractive or ugly, there are options that might be able to restore a good cosmetic appearance without removing the eye. These options include a scleral shell or a cosmetic contact lens.

Scleral Shell

A scleral shell is an ocular prosthesis (see: Prosthesis) that is made extremely thin so that it can fit behind the eyelids and in front of an existing unattractive eye. Scleral shells are fabricated by ocularists, medical health professionals who make artificial eyes. A scleral shell is placed over the unattractive eye between the eyelids. Like an ocular prosthesis, it is fabricated to match the color and appearance of the good eye. A scleral shell would give the best cosmetic result in creating the desired appearance of having eyes that look similar. Unfortunately, a scleral shell is not flexible, and its presence in front of the existing blind eye and behind the eyelids can be uncomfortable to some people. The scleral shell will move as the eye behind it moves. The movement is not as dramatic as the natural eye itself, but it can give an excellent appearance of eye movement.

If the corneal surface, or front covering, of the existing eye is still sensitive, then a scleral shell might produce a foreign body sensation or a feeling that something is in the eye. The patient may not be able to tolerate this feeling of the scleral shell for long periods of time. If the cornea has been damaged and has lost its sensitivity, then the inflexible scleral shell can be very well tolerated.

Charles B. Slonim, MD & Amy Z. Martino MD

Cosmetic Contact Lens

A cosmetic contact lens is a soft contact lens with the image of an eye either painted on the surface or impregnated into the matrix of the soft plastic contact lens material. Because it is a soft contact lens, it is extremely thin and very flexible. The flexibility makes it very comfortable on most eyes. The lens must be centered over the cornea for a good cosmetic result. Blind eyes with distorted corneas from trauma or previous surgeries are not good candidates for cosmetic contact lenses because a contact lens needs a smooth, curved corneal surface to rest on in order to remain centered. Eyes that are not positioned straight ahead, deviated or severely crossed, or turned out are not good candidates for cosmetic contact lenses because the image of the eye would continue to assume the abnormal position of the eye.

Matching the appearance of the good eye with a cosmetic soft contact lens is possible but typically will not be as good as a scleral shell. Nonetheless, with a pair of slightly tinted glasses worn for protection of the good eye, a cosmetic contact lens can offer an excellent cosmetic alternative to surgery.

Surgery

Timing

For the patient, there is rarely a good time to remove an eye. Those rare times usually include when the pain and discomfort of the eye significantly reduce the patient's ability to function in their normal daily activities. The sooner these blind and painful eyes are removed, the faster the patient can get on with his or her life. Delaying the removal of an eye rarely has an effect on the surgical technique or complication rate.

Obviously, the faster an eye with a tumor is removed, the less chance of spread of the tumor to the tissues surrounding the eye in the orbit or to other parts of the body. In cases where an open-globe injury occurred (see: Surgery: Timing: Open Globe Injury), delaying the surgery could have a negative effect on the good, uninjured eye (see: Surgery: Timing: Sympathetic Ophthalmia).

Blind and Painful Eye

A frequent reason that patients give for delaying the removal of a blind and painful eye is hopeful anticipation that future development of new technologies could possibly make the eye see again. There is no surgeon in the world that can predict the future development of an invention or technology that could benefit a patient tomorrow. As of the writing of this book, current technologies such as artificial retinas[11] attempt to recreate visual impulses to the brain that are recognized as a visual image. Even if a radical technology existed, the quality of the vision might not equal that of the good eye. This would create a slight problem for the brain and its ability to interpret that image along with the image from the good eye. If the two images were very different, the brain would simply choose the better vision from the good eye and ignore or suppress the worse image from the bad eye. However, in the case of bilateral (both eyes) blindness, keeping one eye intact and not removing it may give the patient hope for future developments. In all cases, the physical, emotional, or psychological debilitation that the bad eye creates must be weighed against the probabilities that such developments will occur in the near future.

Open-globe Injury

For the surgeon, there are a few unwritten guidelines to follow regarding the timing of removing a blind and painful eye. The discussions regarding the prompt removal of an eye that has suffered an open-globe injury is focused around the prevention of a condition called sympathetic ophthalmia (see: Surgery: Timing: Sympathetic Ophthalmia).

Handling the severely traumatized eye is a true challenge for the ophthalmic surgeon. The surgeon's first priority and concern is to try to repair the damage to the injured eye. The second priority is to try to save the sight in the injured eye. The third priority is to protect the uninjured eye from sympathetic ophthalmia.

The ophthalmic surgeon will always try to repair a severely injured eye as soon as possible after the injury. Surgeons prefer not to remove an injured eye at the first surgery even if it has no light perception. The main reason for this is a psychological one. Most patients with a severely injured eye are not able to understand the gravity of their condition immediately after the injury. Waking up from an initial surgery without an eye can create a tremendous amount of stress and anxiety for the patient. The patient may question whether it was medically or surgically necessary for the eye to be removed. They may wonder if there was any hope of saving the eye. They may question the surgeon's intentions in removing the eye so soon after the injury.

Ophthalmic surgeons will initially make every attempt to repair a severely injured eye even if they believe that there is no hope of saving the sight in that eye. Their goal is to have the patient wake up from the surgery and recognize that they have no sight in the eye. This gives the patient a short period of time to think about their condition and consider their options during a slightly less stressful postoperative period.

Occasionally, when the eye is not surgically reparable, the eye is removed at the initial surgery. If possible, some surgeons will try to obtain a second opinion from another ophthalmic surgeon before removing the eye in this situation, in order to confirm that the eye could not be repaired and needed to be removed.

Sympathetic Ophthalmia

Sympathetic ophthalmia is a condition where the uninjured good eye "sympathizes" with the injured eye and can develop a significant inflammatory response, which can lead to reduced vision and even blindness. By removing the injured eye within seven to ten days of the initial injury, the risk of developing sympathetic ophthalmia in the good eye is reduced to virtually nothing.

The eye is a relatively self-contained organ. The outer coverings of the eye (the white sclera and the clear central cornea) are relatively impervious compared to the surrounding tissues. The internal parts of the eye are not directly connected to any other structures, and the outer sheath of the eye is contiguous with the sheath of the optic nerve. The eye does contain a variety of blood vessels that bring it nourishment and oxygen and remove the metabolic waste products from the eye. The optic nerve contains approximately 1.6 million nerve fibers that connect the photoreceptor cells (i.e., the rods and cones) of the retina to the occipital lobe of the brain. The optic nerve, through which visual images are sent to the brain, is actually an extension of brain tissue. The optic nerve transmits these images, and the brain interprets them as sight.

During severe trauma to the eye where the eyeball is lacerated, some of the internal structures of the eye may escape through the laceration and exit the eye. There are certain parts in the eye such as the iris (the colored portion of the eye), the ciliary body (the part that produces the fluid which fills the inside of the eye), and the choroid (the structure on which the retina lies) that can easily protrude through the open wound of an eyeball injury. As long as these parts remain inside the eye, the body's immune system continues to recognize those parts as part of the eye and part of the person's own body.

If these vital parts leave or exit the eye, the body occasionally declares them as foreign material and no longer part of the person's eye or body. At any time after the injury, the body's immune system may choose to attack these "foreign structures" just as it would try to attack the toxins from a bee sting. This attack is actually an inflammatory response that tries to damage the foreign material so that it can be safely removed from the body by special blood cells of the immune system. Unfortunately, the body's immune system cannot distinguish the difference between the parts of the injured eye that protruded through a laceration and the same normal parts of the good eye, which still remain inside the good eye. Therefore the immune system also attacks these parts of the good eye, causing this condition called sympathetic ophthalmia.

The incidence of sympathetic ophthalmia is rare; it affects between two to five of a thousand open-globe injuries and less than one of a thousand eyes that have had elective eye surgery performed on them. If the injured eye is beyond any hope of recovery of functional vision removed and if it is removed within ten days following the initial injury, then the risk of sympathetic ophthalmia is significantly reduced or eliminated.[12,13] This is one of only a few reasons why a surgeon may suggest removing an injured eye sooner than later. However, if a severely injured eye still has light perception vision or better, then the eye is usually left in place and observed carefully, even if some of the vital parts of the eye, mentioned above, exited the eye.

Sympathetic ophthalmia is treatable if discovered early. The treatment usually requires both steroid eye drops and, frequently, oral steroid medications.

Procedures (The 3 Es)

There are three basic procedures that involve the removal of any combination of the eye, its contents, and its surrounding structures. These are the enucleation, evisceration, and exenteration.

Enucleation

Enucleation is the removal of the eyeball along with all of its internal contents. The first actual report of surgery to remove an eye was described in 1583 by the German ophthalmologist, Dr. George Bartisch.[14,15] The report depicts a method of passing a needle and thread through the eyeball for traction and then passing a curved knife behind the eye to sever the attachments. Anesthesia depended on the amount of induced intoxication (i.e., making the patient extremely drunk). Certainly, this technique is considered barbaric by today's standards; however, as time passed, surgeons continued to advance their knowledge and improve upon their surgical techniques.

An enucleation involves opening the conjunctiva that lies over the surface of the white part of the eye (sclera), detaching the eye muscles that move the eye in different directions and hold the eye in the socket, and finally cutting the optic nerve.

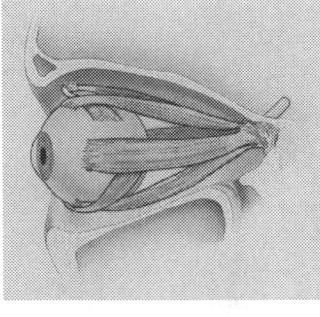
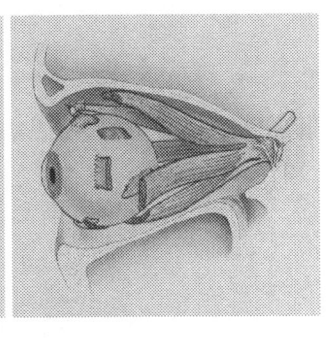

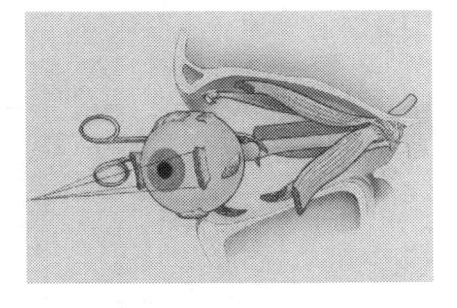

With these supporting structures cut, the eyeball can be safely removed from the socket while leaving all of the surrounding structures, such as the eyelids, conjunctiva, eye muscles and orbital fat, intact.

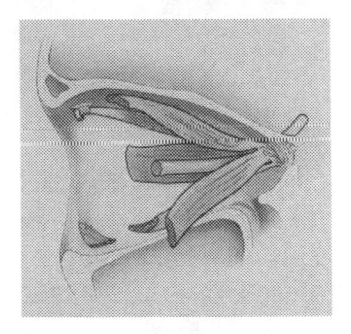

The eye is routinely sent to a pathology laboratory where a pathologist will cut the eye into many slices and look at each slice under the microscope to determine the final condition of each ocular structure.

Once the eye is removed, the physical space that the eye occupied must be replaced. The average volume of an eye is approximately seven milliliters, or the size of a radish. If this volume is not replaced at the time of surgery, the eyelids would sink into the socket. Therefore an orbital implant is inserted into the socket at the time of surgery to replace the lost volume. These implants are available in a number of shapes, sizes, and materials; typically they are spherical in shape. The surgeon will try to implant the largest sized implant that the socket will comfortably hold. The remaining volume loss is replaced by the prosthesis or artificial eye. The larger the implant, the smaller (and lighter weight) the prosthesis will eventually be.

Today, there are basically two kinds of orbital implants that are inserted into the socket after an eye is removed: those that are porous and can be integrated with the prosthesis and those that are nonporous and cannot be integrated with the prosthesis. The nonporous implants are made of an acrylic or silicone material. These spherical implants look like large marbles and come in a variety of diameters.

Once the nonporous implant is inserted into the socket, the eye muscles that were detached from the eye are sutured together in front of the implant. This holds the implant in place, preventing it from protruding forward. The two vertical muscles (superior rectus and inferior rectus) are sewn together, as are the two horizontal muscles (medial rectus and lateral rectus). These muscles are still capable of moving when the other good eye moves. Two or three more layers of orbital tissues are then sewn in front of the muscles. The socket will eventually create a fibrous layer of scar tissue around the implant. The last layer to be sewn together is the conjunctiva, which is the transparent mucous membrane that covers the surface of the white part of the eye and lines the inside of the eyelids. The conjunctiva contains all of the blood vessels that make an eye red when an eye infection or inflammation exists. When the surgery is completed and if the eyelids are opened, the resulting appearance is that of a pink wall. This pink wall is the final layer of the conjunctiva.

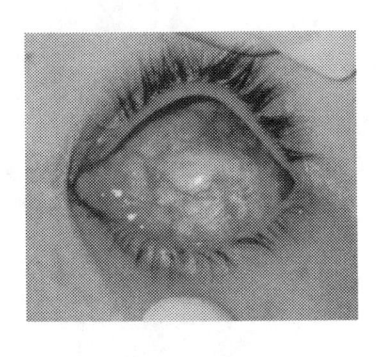

Immediately after surgery, the surgeon will place a clear, slightly concave (like half of an almond shell), plastic conformer between the eyelids and in front of the pink wall to keep the socket shaped and the eyelids curved. Eventually the conformer will be replaced by the prosthesis or artificial eye. When the eye muscles move, some of this movement is transferred to this wall of conjunctiva. This movement is eventually transferred to the artificial eye. Most patients will wear a patch to cover the eyelids and conformer until the artificial eye is in place.

Natural-Iris Conformers (from Porex Surgical, Inc.) are conformers that have an image of an iris and pupil incorporated on the surface. They are available in six iris colors (blue, blue-gray, green hazel, brown hazel, medium brown, and dark brown). These conformers can be used in place of clear conformers immediately after surgery, which allows the patient to heal comfortably without requiring an eye patch during the postoperative period prior to fitting a custom-made prosthesis.

Porous implants are made of a couple of special materials that contain thousands of microscopic channels and pores, like a sponge. These implants, however, are rigid like the nonporous implants and are not actually soft like a sponge. The two most common materials that the porous implants are made of are high-density polyethylene (e.g., MEDPOR from Porex Surgical, Inc.) and hydroxyapatite (e.g., Bio-Eye from Integrated Orbital Implants, Inc.). These are also referred to as integrateable implants because they can be directly attached to the prosthesis through a connecting device (i.e., motility peg). This integration offers better movement of the prosthesis or artificial eye after surgery.

There are two special features of the porous implants. The first feature is that the eye muscles that were detached from the enucleated (removed) eye can be sewn directly onto the implant in the relatively same positions from where they where removed.

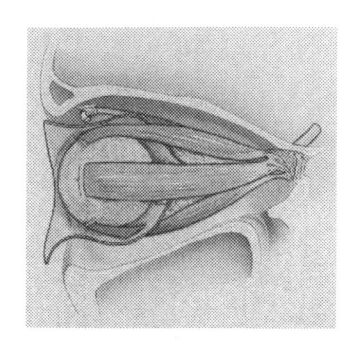

Some of the porous implants (e.g., hydroxyapatite) are wrapped in a covering material before they are implanted; this makes it easier for the surgeon to insert the implant and also improves the socket's ability to hold the implant in place. The wrapping material may be synthetic and commercially prepared, or it may come from tissues obtained from other parts of the body (e.g., a tendon or fascia). The muscles are sewn onto the wrapping material. Some high-density polyethylene implants (MEDPOR) have preplaced holes and tunnels where the sutures can be easily passed. This material can be inserted without the need of a wrapping material.

The second feature of these implants is that the blood vessels from the eye socket can get into the pores and channels of the porous material and grow directly inside the implant. This process is known as vascularization, which essentially allows the implant to become a living part of the socket with its own blood supply. After the muscles are attached to the implant, two or three more layers of tissue are then sewn in front of the muscles just as with the nonporous implants. The last layer to be sewn together is also the conjunctiva layer, resulting in the same pink wall appearance.

Immediately after surgery with an integrateable implant, the surgeon will also place a clear plastic conformer or Natural-Iris Conformer behind the eyelids and in front of the pink wall.

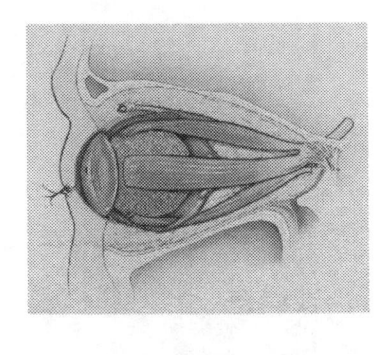

Eventually this conformer will also be replaced by the artificial eye. When the eye muscles move, there is more movement transferred to the pink wall. It takes about six months to a year after the operation for the porous implant to become completely vascularized. That means that the implant is completely filled with blood vessels that have grown into it from the surrounding orbital tissues.

The vast majority of enucleation surgeries are performed as an outpatient in either a hospital outpatient department or a free-standing outpatient surgery facility. Some patients may require hospitalization and overnight observation depending on their general health conditions. The surgery is performed under general anesthesia, where the patient is asleep for the entire surgery. The surgery can be performed under local anesthesia with sedation, if necessary.

The postoperative course following an enucleation will differ from patient to patient. The amount of postoperative discomfort or pain differs depending on the complexity of the surgery and the sensitivity of the remaining orbital tissues. It also depends on the patient's tolerance for pain. Some patients may only require an over-the-counter analgesic such as Extra-Strength Tylenol, but others may require prescription narcotics. In either case, the need for analgesics is typically short-lived; lasting a few days to a week. By far, the vast majority of patient who go into surgery with a painful eye leave the recovery room with less pain than before the surgery.

Postoperative nausea can also exist for a day or two after surgery, but it can be controlled by prescription medications if necessary. The majority of the postoperative discomfort occurs when the eye is moving; this is probably due to the rearrangement of the eye muscles at the time of surgery. When the good eye moves, so do the redirected eye muscles in the enucleated socket. However, the muscles are pulling in slightly different directions than they had been preoperatively.

The postoperative care required by the patient following an enucleation differs from surgeon to surgeon. The patient routinely receives written postoperative instructions along with required medication prescriptions prior to discharge from the surgery facility. Some surgeons may prescribe postoperative oral antibiotics for up to a week after surgery to prevent infection. Other surgeons may choose instead to give the antibiotics intravenously before the surgery starts. Some surgeons will prescribe an oral steroid, such as Prednisone, for a few days after surgery to reduce the inflammation associated with the surgery; this is more common when the porous implants are used.

Almost all patients will be asked to use a topical ophthalmic antibiotic ointment after surgery. This ointment will either be a pure antibiotic ointment or a combination of an antibiotic mixed with a steroid. About a quarter inch of the ointment is placed between the eyelids in front of the clear plastic conformer. When the eyelids are closed, the body temperature melts the ointment and allows it to spread evenly around the conformer. The ointment is usually used once or twice a day for a week or two. A clean cotton eye patch is taped over the eyelids to keep foreign material from contaminating the socket. The patch is changed on a daily basis and is usually worn until the prosthesis is made.

After the socket has had a chance to heal, the patient is then sent to the ocularist for the initial fitting and fabrication of the prosthesis. The healing process takes between three and eight weeks, depending on the surgeon's postoperative protocol and the patient's postoperative course. The tissues of the socket need to be free of inflammation and free of any residual swelling so that an appropriately sized prosthesis can be designed.

Once a porous implant is vascularized, a small titanium peg can be screwed into the implant through the pink wall.

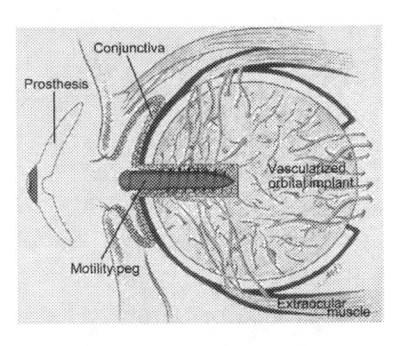

Some porous implants require that a hollow, threaded sleeve be screwed into the implant. A removable peg is placed into the center of the sleeve.

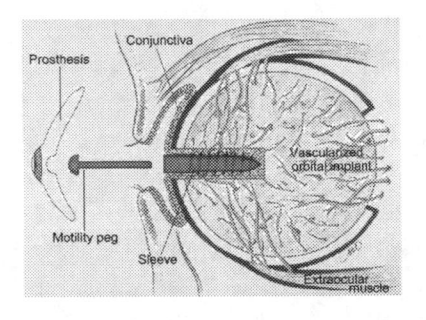

This can frequently be done in the surgeon's office or at an outpatient surgery facility with local anesthesia. The end of the peg will stick out a few millimeters from the pink wall. A special prosthesis with a small dimple in the back of it is made by the ocularist; the peg fits into the dimple. As the eye muscles move, the porous implant moves, and therefore, the peg moves. This movement is eventually transferred to the artificial eye. The movement is considerably more with the peg than without it. This technique of enucleation with implantation of an integrateable implant offers the patient the most movement of their prosthesis. There are, however, a few additional postoperative complications specifically associated with the peg (see: Surgery: Complications of Surgery). Because the insertion of a motility peg is only meant to enhance the movement of the prosthesis, it is typically considered a cosmetic procedure by most insurance companies. Therefore the motility pegging of an implant is typically an out-of-pocket expense.

Evisceration

An evisceration is quite different from an enucleation. An evisceration is a surgical procedure where the eye is surgically opened, and only the internal contents of the eye—including the iris, lens, retina, and other internal parts—are totally removed.

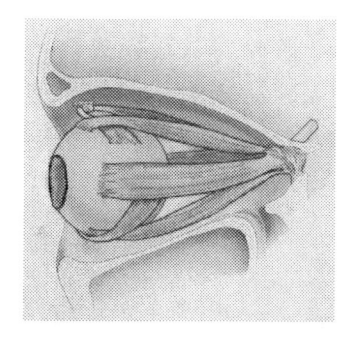

The first evisceration performed as a routine procedure was done by Noyes in 1874.[15] The white shell (sclera) and sometimes the clear cornea of the eye are left intact in the socket with the muscles still attached to the sclera. The only similarity to the enucleation is that a space-occupying spherical implant must also be inserted into the socket to replace the loss of volume caused by removing the contents of the eye. In eviscerations, however, the implant is inserted into the hollowed sclera, and the sclera is sutured closed around the implant. A layer of conjunctiva is sewn in front of the closed scleral shell. Therefore the final appearance after an evisceration (i.e., the pink wall of conjunctiva) will be similar to that after an enucleation.

The surgeon also has the option of using either a porous or nonporous implant. If a porous implant is chosen, then small windows are cut into the scleral shell to allow blood vessels from the orbit to grow into the pores and channels of the implant.

Because the muscles remain attached to the original shell of the eye, the movement of the implant is almost as good as the original eye. This movement is transferred to the pink wall, which is then transferred to the prosthesis. The porous implants can be pegged six to twelve months later for better motility, if the patient desires.

The postoperative care following an evisceration is almost identical to that of an enucleation. Postoperative swelling and discomfort tends to be a little more after eviscerations than after enucleations. This is felt to be due to the fact that an empty scleral shell remains in the socket even though it is "filled" with an implant. The socket reacts to this scleral shell with more inflammation than when the entire eye is removed during an enucleation.

The use of postoperative antibiotics, steroids, pain, and possibly nausea medications is similar to that after enucleation surgery and will differ from surgeon to surgeon as well as from patient to patient.

Evisceration surgery is frequently the surgery of choice in the situation where the eye has suffered a severe internal infection, known as an endophthalmitis. In an endophthalmitis, the internal tissues of the eye are infected with bacteria, viruses, or fungi, and the inside of the eye frequently contains pus. Even after aggressive treatment with topical antibiotics, systemic antibiotics, and even antibiotics injected directly into the eye, an eye which has suffered an endophthalmitis can eventually go blind with no light perception. In this situation, the infected contents of the eye need to be removed in order to resolve the infection. The surgeon may choose to eviscerate the eye but not insert an implant during the initial evisceration surgery. This is done specifically to allow the infection to completely drain and resolve before inserting an implant, and it prevents any residual infection from getting trapped inside the closed scleral shell with an implant inside of it. In these cases, the scleral shell is left open for seven to ten days. Some surgeons will place a small amount of packing in the scleral shell to keep the edges of the sclera open. After the surgeon is confident that there are no signs of the initial infection, he or she will then insert a secondary implant, porous or nonporous, at a second surgery. The final result is similar to a primary evisceration surgery where the implant is inserted at the time of the initial surgery. The pink wall of conjunctiva is the final layer that is seen between the eyelids. A temporary clear conformer or Natural Iris Conformer is placed between the eyelids while awaiting the prosthesis.

Similar to enucleation surgery, after the socket has had a chance to heal, the patient is then sent to the ocularist for the initial fitting and fabrication of the prosthesis. This can take between three and eight weeks, depending on the surgeon's postoperative protocol and the patient's postoperative course. The tissues of the socket need to be free of inflammation and free of any residual swelling so that an appropriate sized prosthesis can be designed.

Exenteration

An exenteration is a procedure that is typically reserved for the removal of malignant cancers of the orbit. These cancers may have originated from the eyelids or the eye itself but have unfortunately spread to the surrounding tissues of the orbit. Malignant tumors can originate from the structures that surround the eye such as the lacrimal (tear) gland or even the sinuses; these tumors can eventually spread to the eye.

An exenteration is a disfiguring surgery. Although there are no historic records that specifically describe the first reported exenteration, many of the early enucleations included the removal of surrounding orbital tissues such as eye muscles, conjunctiva, and orbital fat and fascia, which would be classified as partial exenterations. The surgery not only involves removing the eye but also involves removing the eyelids, eye muscles, and the surrounding orbital structures such as the lacrimal glands and orbital fat. If the cancer has spread to the orbital bones, then portions of the bones may have to be removed, which will expose the sinuses that border the orbit. The patient is left with an empty socket that appears as a small, open cavity in the front of the face where the eye used to be.

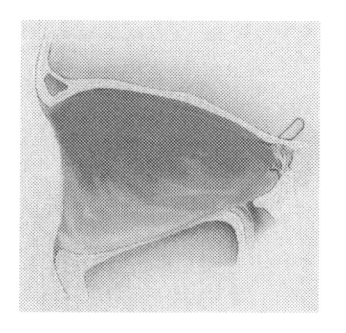

The exposed bones of the orbital walls inside of the socket are usually covered with a skin graft, which is usually taken from the skin of the upper thigh.

The postoperative care of the exenterated socket requires a lot more work than either an enucleation or an evisceration. Postoperative care is also required of the site where the skin graft came from (donor site). The final healing process may take three to four months before a prosthesis can be fit.

Exenterated patients typically do not have as much postoperative pain or nausea as enucleated or eviscerated patients. This is probably related to the fact that most of the sensory nerves are removed at the time of the exenteration. Postoperative oral antibiotics are usually prescribed for a week or two after the surgery. Usually the socket is filled with sterile gauze that is left in place for up to a week. The socket is then patched and left untouched for the first week; there is really nothing for the patient to do with the socket for the first week after surgery.

The donor site from where the skin graft came will require the most attention in the immediate postoperative period. Because only the most superficial layer of skin is required, the remaining surface looks like a bad skin abrasion (e.g., a rug burn) in the shape of a rectangle. This rectangle will vary in size depending on the amount of skin required to cover the socket. Many surgeons cover the donor site with a clear adhesive dressing that remains in place until it falls off on its own, usually four to five days. Once the adhesive dressing falls off, the skin surface usually has a lot of dried blood over it. This can be gently removed with warm, wet compresses. Patients should avoid rubbing the healing donor site to prevent bleeding. Once the dressing is off, the donor site can be left uncovered and open to the air, and antibiotic ointments or creams may be prescribed.

By this time (approximately one week after surgery), the patch and socket packing will have been removed by the surgeon during one of the postoperative visits. The skin graft will have a lot of dried blood and a number of small blisters that the surgeon may or may not open and drain. This first cleaning of the socket is always done by the surgeon or possibly an assistant. After this, the patient or caretaker may be asked to routinely or occasionally clean the socket at home. This may only require removing the larger, loose pieces of dried blood and secretions. Some surgeons may suggest using a diluted hydrogen peroxide solution to keep the socket clean. Other surgeons may require weekly visits to the office within the first month or so and perform all cleaning themselves. Once the graft and socket have healed, the patient is sent to an ocularist or anaplastologist that creates orbital prostheses.

An orbital prosthesis is a large, sculpted acrylic form that fills the empty socket. This three-dimensional form contains artificially created upper and lower eyelids with eyelashes that do not move and an artificial eye which also does not move. It is custom fitted to each individual socket, and it is held in place by a few different methods. A skin adhesive at the edge of the prosthesis can be used to secure the prosthesis to the skin of the outer rim of the socket. Occasionally magnets can also be used to hold the prosthesis in place after a circular frame of magnets is inserted just inside the outer rim of the socket. Some orbital prostheses are attached directly to the frame of a pair of glasses. A well-fit orbital prosthesis with a pair of protective glasses over it can look amazingly similar to the good eye on the other side.

Complications of Surgery

As with any surgical procedure, a 100 percent successful outcome can never be guaranteed by the surgeon. However, the three E surgeries (enucleation, evisceration, and exenteration) have excellent postoperative success rates. As with any surgical procedure, identical procedures performed by the same surgeon on the same day on two different patients with the same condition may have two completely different surgical outcomes. Individual patients heal differently, and postoperative conditions may have different effects on the healing processes of different patients. Obviously the surgeon wants to have the same successful outcome on all patients, but the surgical outcome of a traumatized eye is directly related to the nature, extent, and severity of the injury; no two injured eyes behave the same.

The final postoperative appearance after a very successful surgery with the best manufactured prosthesis will be perceived differently by different people. What looks good to the surgeon, his or her staff, and others may not look good to the patient.

Surgical complications are usually divided into three categories: those that occur during the surgery (intraoperative), those that occur in the early postoperative period (within a few weeks) and those that occur in the late postoperative period (months to years after surgery).

Intraoperative

The most feared complication of any ophthalmic surgery is the worsening or loss of vision that existed before surgery. Obviously with enucleation, evisceration, and exenteration surgeries, vision is not a concern of the surgeon because it has been predetermined that the eye is going to be removed. The main intraoperative complication that the ophthalmic surgeon faces with these surgeries is excessive bleeding that becomes difficult to control. With excessive bleeding comes swelling and distortion of the surrounding anatomical structures, which can make the surgery significantly more difficult.

Excessive bleeding or swelling at the time of surgery can force a surgeon to insert a smaller than desired implant into the socket since the swelling will not allow the larger, more appropriate sized implant to fit. Inserting a larger implant into a swollen socket could risk an extrusion of the implant in the immediate postoperative period. When the swelling eventually resolves, the socket may show the undesired effects of volume loss because a smaller than desired implant had to be inserted. This volume loss, where the eyelids appear sunken in, can be compensated for with either a large-sized prosthesis or possibly surgically exchanging the implant for a larger one at some future date.

On rare occasions, usually in severe trauma, an implant cannot be inserted at the time of the initial surgery. In these situations the socket is allowed to settle down and heal for a few weeks, and then a secondary implant is inserted at a second surgery.

Early Postoperative

The development of an early postoperative infection is always a major concern of the surgeon. Infections can delay healing and possibly ruin the desired effects of surgery. Preoperative prevention of an infection begins in the operating room with the use of standard sterile surgical techniques throughout the surgery. Occasionally antibiotics are given intravenously either before or during the surgery. Postoperative prevention of infection is usually the responsibility of the patient. Frequently the surgeon will prescribe oral antibiotics for up to a week, and topical antibiotics in the form of ointments or drops are almost always used directly on the surgical sites. The patient needs to keep the surgical area clean and avoid situations where unwanted debris or dirt could get into the socket. The patient should thoroughly wash his or her hands before treating the socket with ointment or drops and changing the patch.

The most common postoperative finding after enucleation and evisceration surgeries is swelling of the eyelids. (In cases of exenteration, the eyelids are removed during, and so this is not an issue.) The amount of swelling depends on the difficulties encountered during the surgery and the length of the surgery, but it is also related to the way that the patient's orbital tissues react to the surgery. Some surgeons will allow their patients to place cold or iced compresses on the eyelids during the first forty-eight to seventy two hours after surgery starting on the day following removal of the patch. The cold compresses reduce and prevent further swelling. After this period, warm compresses are used to help reduce the existing swelling that is present in the tissues. The warm compresses can be continued until the swelling has completely gone away.

Another common postoperative finding is called chemosis (pronounced *keem-ó-sis*). Chemosis refers to a swollen conjunctiva. Sometimes the conjunctiva becomes so swollen that it will push the conformer out from behind the eyelids. When the conjunctiva is that swollen, the conformer cannot be put back in until the conjunctival swelling has gone away. Without the conformer, the chemosis protrudes between the eyelids. Frequently the chemosis is associated with blood that has become trapped in the conjunctiva; this is called a subconjunctival hemorrhage because the blood or hemorrhage is actually trapped under the surface of the conjunctiva. When the conjunctiva sticks out between the eyelids, it can look pretty strange and unattractive. However, this condition is harmless and will go away on its own over time; severe chemosis takes a couple of weeks to go away. Chemosis can delay the initial fitting of the prosthesis. As soon as the conformer can be placed behind the eyelids, it should be put there in order to maintain the shape of the socket.

Occasionally surgical wounds that have been sutured together may separate. This is known as a wound dehiscence. Sometimes the patient is brought back to the operating room to repair the open wound. Other times the open wound is left alone and allowed to continue through the healing process for repair at a later time. In the case of enucleations and eviscerations, wound dehiscence can result in the extrusion of the implant that was placed in the socket or scleral shell, respectively. Immediate repair of these wounds is usually necessary.

Enucleation and evisceration patients will frequently experience a day or two of postoperative nausea, sometimes vomiting. This is usually controlled with medications.

Postoperative pain varies considerably from patient to patient and from surgery to surgery. Many factors contribute to the level of discomfort and pain experienced by an individual patient: the condition of the structures that surround the eye (e.g., orbital fractures), the difficulty of the surgery, the sensitivity of the remaining orbital nerves, and the pain tolerance of the patient. Some patients may require only over-the-counter analgesics, but others may require potent narcotics (e.g., Percocet, Vicodin).

Bruising of the eyelids and skin around the orbit is very common after surgery. This is expected and not considered a complication. Blood-tinged pink tears can occur for a few days or even as long as a week. Patients who take blood thinners (aspirin, Plavix, Coumadin, etc.) for other medical conditions prior to surgery can expect more bruising than those patients who do not take blood thinners. When possible, blood thinners will be discontinued prior to performing surgery.

Enucleation and evisceration surgeries do not involve the lacrimal gland. Therefore tears are still produced after these surgeries and fill the space between the eyelids and the pink wall. These tears continue to lubricate the conformer initially and then the prosthesis later. A healthy tear film keeps the prosthesis looking shiny and appearing more realistic. Exenteration surgery removes the lacrimal gland, and therefore tear production is permanently discontinued.

It is not uncommon for secretions from the operative site such as tears, serum, or even blood to stick to the lashes or the skin and form crusts and scabs. When the lids are closed for long periods of time (e.g., during sleep), these crusts might cause the lids to stick together. Warm, wet compresses placed against the eyelids can help loosen or even melt these dried secretions, which can then be gently wiped away. It is essential that the lid margins be kept free of these secretions because they can serve as a feeding ground for a variety of microorganisms such as bacteria.

Late Postoperative

Late surgical complications usually involve the socket. Chronic socket pain is rare but can occur; the cause of the pain is not always obvious, and the actual source is frequently difficult to find. The pain can be related to damage sustained at the time of the original injury and damage to orbital structures as a result of the original medical condition that necessitated the removal of the eye. Pain may be related to irritated nerve endings that result from the surgery. Every surgical procedure makes physical and structural changes in the original anatomy of the tissues on which are being operated. Even the smallest piece of scar tissue that inadvertently touches a sensory nerve can cause chronic pain and discomfort in a socket without an eye. Rough edges on prostheses have also been known to cause late postoperative discomfort.

Extrusions of the implants in enucleation and evisceration surgeries can occur even after uneventful and uncomplicated surgery. The surgeon uses many techniques during surgery to ensure that the implant remains in place after surgery. Unfortunately, on occasion the socket will try to push the implant out of the socket over time. This is usually a gradual process over weeks or months. The patient will start to notice that their prosthesis is not fitting well or is slowly pushing forward. Surgery may be required to either reposition the implant or remove and replace the implant with one of a different size or shape. The porous implants are less likely to extrude from the socket than the nonporous ones because the muscles have been attached directly to the porous implants or its wrapping material. The nonporous implants have the potential to extrude from the socket even many years after the initial surgery to implant them.

As with any surgical site, localized changes of the surrounding tissues can occur that make the socket no longer capable of holding or retaining a prosthesis. Further surgeries may be required to repair the socket so that the prosthesis can be fit and worn properly. An incompetent socket may occur in many different ways. One of the most common causes of an incompetent socket is a sagging lower lid, referred to as a lower lid ectropion. An ectropion makes it difficult for the lower lid to support the weight of the prosthesis, causing the prosthesis to fall out with minimal manipulation or movement.

Socket scarring related to the initial trauma or surgery might prevent the prosthesis from properly positioning itself in the socket. Scarring of the conjunctiva is referred to as a symblepharon. Dividing or removing the scar tissue during another surgery might allow the prosthesis to fit better; surgical grafting may be required to prevent the scars from returning. A small piece of mucous membrane taken from the inside of the lower lip is frequently used as a grafting material because this tissue very closely resembles the structure and function of the conjunctiva. Amniotic membrane can also be used as a grafting material.

Occasionally, conjunctival scarring on the inside of the socket can cause an eyelid to turn in. This is called an entropion. When an eyelid is turned inward, the lashes will touch the prosthesis and sometimes get stuck to the surface of the prosthesis. Correcting an entropion requires surgery to rotate the eyelid back into its normal position.

Drooping of the upper lid, referred to as a ptosis (pronounced *tóe sis*), is also a common late complication that can occur as a normal part of the aging process or after any type of eye surgery (cataract surgery, glaucoma surgery, etc.). A ptosis can also occur as a direct result of trauma to the socket. There are many surgical procedures available to repair a droopy upper eyelid.

Conjunctivitis, commonly referred to as pink eye, can also occur in the socket even though there is no eye present. The thin mucous membrane of the conjunctiva covers the back side of the eyelids and the front side of the socket (the pink wall). The small space behind a prosthesis is dark, warm, and moist—a perfect environment for microorganisms such as bacteria or viruses to grow and multiply. The same microorganisms that cause a conjunctivitis in a normal eye can cause infection in the socket without an eye. Eye doctors will typically prescribe antibiotic drops if they suspect that the infection is caused by bacteria.

The socket conjunctiva can also be affected by allergies just like the conjunctiva of the normal eye. Allergic conjunctivitis is common in people who suffer from allergies. The most common symptom of allergic conjunctivitis is itchy eyes. Itching can also occur in the socket of a person who has allergies. Anti-allergy eye drops are prescribed to reduce the itching and irritation caused by this condition.

An inflammatory reaction on the inside of the upper eyelid known as giant papillary conjunctivitis can cause the prosthesis to become uncomfortable. In this condition, small elevations or bumps (papillae) occur on the inside surface (conjunctiva) of the upper eyelid. These papillae cause an increased production of mucous that sticks to the prosthesis and makes the socket uncomfortable, especially when blinking.

Inside the normal socket, orbital fat surrounds the eyeball, cushioning the eye as it moves. The fat also cushions the eye when a person rubs their eye, pushing it backwards into the socket. It remains in the socket following enucleation and evisceration surgeries, however most of the fat is removed during exenteration surgery. Placement of the implants at the time of these surgeries is meant to maintain the original volume of the socket. Even if the appropriate-sized implant is placed, there is a chance that the remaining fat changes causing its volume to decrease; this is known as fat necrosis. Fat necrosis directly reduces the volume of fat and causes the eyelids and prosthesis to sink in because of this volume loss. The sinking in of the prosthesis is referred to as enophthalmos. Occasionally this enophthalmos has to be treated in order to maintain the integrity of the socket. Volume replacement fillers such as fat from other areas of the body or synthetic volume replacement implants (e.g., MEDPOR Enophthalmos Wedge) are frequently utilized to increase the volume of the socket. Occasionally the fat volume can be replaced by taking fat from another part of the body (e.g., the flank or "love handles") and transplanting it into the socket. This graft is referred to as a dermis-fat graft and contains a thin layer of the dermis, which remains attached to the fat. The dermis is the tissue layer just below the surface of the skin. Unfortunately, even after successful dermis-fat graft surgery, the newly transplanted fat can eventually undergo necrosis, leading to repeated volume loss.

Late socket infections are rare but can occur, especially with the porous implants. This is because of the porous composition of these implants. If bacteria find their way into the pores or channels of a porous implant, the bacteria can eventually multiply to the extent that a chronic socket infection occurs.

Two common late complications associated with porous implants are exposure of the implant through the pink wall and development of conjunctival growths around the motility peg. Both of these complications are handled surgically.

An exposed implant occurs when the conjunctival wall in front of it becomes extremely thin, eventually uncovering the actual implant material. This issue usually requires surgically closing the tissues over it; it may also require the use of grafts to prevent the exposure from reoccurring. A porous implant that is chronically exposed is at risk for an infection. Occasionally such an implant may have to be removed and replaced with another porous implant. Some surgeons will only implant a nonporous implant after removing an infected porous implant.

A granuloma is a growth of abnormal conjunctival tissue associated with inflammation, and it appears as a soft pink stalk of tissue between the eyelids. These growths tend to develop around the motility pegs associated with the porous implants, but they can also occur on the pink wall even when there is no motility peg in place. They can be removed surgically under local anesthesia but have a tendency to reoccur. Occasionally, the motility peg has to be removed and left out indefinitely.

There are other potential problems that can occur with the motility pegs used to integrate the porous implants with the prosthesis. After an enucleation or evisceration where a porous implant has been placed, six to twelve months must pass before a motility peg is inserted into the front of the implant. This allows the socket time for the surrounding blood vessels to grow into the implant and vascularize the implant. A vascularized porous implant essentially becomes a living part of the socket with its own blood supply. Surgeons will wait until the implant is well vascularized before inserting a motility peg. Some pegs can be screwed directly into the implant material, and others require the insertion of a sleeve into which the motility peg is placed. Sleeves are screwed into the implant material and have a small central tunnel for the stem of the peg to slide into.

A successful integration of the implant with the prosthesis depends on a variety of factors including the strength of the implant material, the integrity of the socket and surrounding tissues, and the size and shape of the prosthesis. Motility pegs associated with sleeves can loosen over time, which can create future problems. Occasionally the sleeves may have to be removed and replaced. Sometimes the pegs may need to be exchanged or removed permanently. Pegs that are screwed directly into an implant without the need for a sleeve do not have these same potential complications.

Depending on the amount of prosthesis movement with and without a motility peg, the surgeon and the patient may choose not to keep the motility peg in place. As with all medical and surgical procedures, the benefits of having the motility peg (the increased movement of the prosthesis) must outweigh the risks of possible or ongoing complications (granulomas). Many surgeons implant porous implants and only peg a small percentage of their patients that have such implants. The option to insert a motility peg always exists as long as the porous implant remains in the socket.

A crusty prosthesis is considered another late complication. It is not uncommon for natural secretions from the socket such as tears or mucous to stick to the prosthesis. The tear film is made up of a three-layer composition. By volume, the thickest layer is the middle layer of water, which is produced by the main and accessory lacrimal glands located in both the socket and the conjunctiva. The inner layer is a layer of mucous, which is produced by special cells (goblet cells) of the conjunctiva. The outer layer is a thin film of oil, which is produced by special glands (meibomian glands) located in the eyelids. This oily layer is meant to prevent the water layer from evaporating.

The function of the tear film is to wet the surface of the prosthesis with each blink just as it would have kept the surface of the eye moist. This wet surface adds to the natural appearance and luster of the prosthesis. Dried secretions and crusts can stick to the man-made, synthetic surface of the prosthesis, and they can cause a lack of luster of the prosthesis and allow more tears to accumulate on top of existing crusts. Bacteria can use these crusts as a source of nutrition, which can result in chronic infections. These secretions and deposits on the prosthesis need to be removed as often as possible in order to prolong the life of the prosthesis (see: Prosthesis: Care and Handling).

Socket Reconstruction

Fortunately, most of the socket abnormalities causing an incompetent socket listed under late complications of surgery are surgically reparable. As with any surgical procedure, timing of the procedure is essential to the eventual success of the operation. The socket should be stable, which means that its physical condition hasn't changed in a few months. Operating prematurely on a progressively changing socket lowers the likelihood of success. The surgeon will choose the best time to operate on an incompetent socket to give it the best chance of healing appropriately so that a prosthesis can be fit properly.

Socket reconstructions can require significant surgical manipulations in order to reestablish the cosmetic appearance of the socket. Such reconstructions may only need repositioning or repair of the eyelids; skin or mucous membrane grafting may or may not be required. Other reconstructions may require surgical procedures deeper into the socket at the level of the implant. Some may necessitate rearrangement of the bones of the orbit.

A shrinking socket may require conformers or symblepharon rings to stretch the inside of the socket so that the prosthesis can be held in place. These conformers may have to be sewn into place for a few weeks or months in order to accomplish the desired reformation of the conjunctival fornices. Conformers and symblepharon rings are available in different shapes and sizes. The surgeon will choose the appropriate one for each socket.

Upper eyelids are known to droop after any kind of eye surgery. This can also occur after enucleation or evisceration surgeries. The surgeries that were performed prior to removing the eye often may have already caused an upper lid to droop (ptosis). Ptosis that follows direct trauma will occasionally resolve on its own, with the eyelid returning to its origin position before the trauma; however, this can take many months to resolve. Most surgeons will wait until there is no change in the position of the upper lid before they consider surgery. The surgeon's choice of operation varies depending on the condition of the eyelid. It is also dependant on the strength of the muscle responsible for raising the eyelid.

When the replacement volumes of the orbital implant plus the prosthesis do not fill the original volume of the eye in the socket, then the socket may start to have some subtle or noticeable physical features. A common feature found in patients with a loss of volume is called a superior sulcus deformity, which is a physical depression or hollowness that is found in the upper eyelid just below the eyebrow. It is typically caused by a loss of orbital volume of the contents of the orbit. There are a variety of different surgeries that can be performed to try to fill out the superior sulcus; the goal is to increase the soft tissue volume of the socket that fills out the superior sulcus. Some of these surgeries include removing the orbital implant and replacing it with a larger one. Inserting a second implant (e.g., a MEDPOR Enophthalmos Wedge) under the existing implant can also increase the volume inside the socket. Because the loss of volume is frequently attributed to a reduced volume of orbital fat, a dermis-fat graft can be used to restore the original volume of fat. Dermatologic fillers (e.g., Restylane, JuveDerm) can also be injected into the sulcus to fill it out. Unfortunately, these fillers are only temporary and require repeat injections every six to ten months. In some selected patients, the removal of excessive skin from the upper eyelid on the opposite side may restore the symmetry of both upper eyelids and make the superior sulcus deformity less noticeable.

The structure and position of the lower eyelids can also change when a prosthesis is present in the socket. The eyeball is supported inside the socket by a number of soft tissue structures, including muscles and fascia. A prosthesis is a relatively small but freely movable device whose weight can place a downward force on the lower eyelid. Over time this weight can slowly stretch the supporting tendons of the lower eyelid, causing the lid to sag. If the lower eyelid sags too much, the prosthesis will not fit appropriately and can possibly fall out.

Surgically tightening the lower eyelid can reestablish the integrity of the socket and prevent the prosthesis from falling out.

One of the most difficult postoperative complications that a surgeon has to deal with is socket contracture. Contraction or shrinking of the soft tissues of the socket can be the result of the original condition or trauma that caused the eye to be removed, or of multiple surgeries that the socket and the eye experienced. It can also be a result of certain treatments such as radiation therapy that might have been required to treat the original condition in the eye or orbit.

Most contracted sockets are unable to hold a prosthesis. The majority of surgeries to repair a contracted socket are performed with the goal of getting a prosthesis to fit properly and look similar to the other side. Scarring within the soft tissues typically causes the contraction, which can exist in any one or all of the orbital tissues including the skin of the eyelids, the conjunctiva, or the tissues deeper in the socket. Depending on the quality and quantity of the tissues that are contracted, repairing a contracted socket frequently takes more than one surgery. Repairing a contracted socket frequently requires grafting with soft tissues taken from other parts of the body. For example, when additional skin is required, thin and hairless skin may be taken from behind an ear, from on top of a collar bone, or from the opposite eyelid. When more conjunctiva is needed for the inside of the socket, a piece of mucous membrane from inside the lower lip can be used. One of the problems that a surgeon faces when repairing abnormal scar tissue is that the surgery to repair it creates new scar tissue. This new scar tissue can cause the final results of the surgery to fail.

Extrusions of the implants in enucleation and evisceration surgeries can occur even after uncomplicated surgery (see: Complications of Surgery: Late Postoperative). Extrusions where the implant slowly works it way out of the socket are rare, especially with the porous implants because the muscles are attached directly to it. A more frequent socket complication is the situation where the porous implant remains in position, but its surface becomes exposed; this can occur from a variety of reasons where the pink wall becomes so thin that it opens up and exposes the surface of the implant, and it can lead to an infection because the implant is now open to the environment and not completely covered. If the porous implant has not become completely vascularized, surgeries to cover the exposed area are more difficult because the tissue that will be used by the surgeon to cover the area of exposure will not have blood vessels to help in the healing process. The surgical techniques needed to cover the exposed implant depend on the size of the area of exposure, the vascularization of the implant, and the condition of the surrounding tissues (usually conjunctiva). Frequently a mucous membrane graft taken from the lower lip can be used to cover an exposed implant. In more difficult cases, especially with infected implants, the implant may have to be removed and replaced.

The ability to open and close and blink the eyelids around a prosthesis in a symmetrical fashion as the good eye is completely dependent on the condition of the eyelid muscles that are specifically responsible for those actions and the nerves that control the actions of those muscles. Injury or damage to those muscles or nerves may directly affect eyelid movement. Any decrease in blinking or elevation of the upper eyelid (e.g., retraction) or drooping of the lower eyelid can create a condition commonly referred to as a prosthetic stare. In a prosthetic stare, the prosthesis appears to be gazing directly at someone or something, and looks unnatural. A prosthetic stare can also occur if the eye muscles in the socket are unable to move the prosthesis well. When a prosthesis does not move well, it basically remains in one position while the other eye moves normally, which can become very obvious to the observer.

Pediatric Anophthalmos

Socket Development

As mentioned above (see: Causes: Birth Defects), when an infant or toddler is missing an eye due to a congenital defect or surgery, the surgeon must not only focus on the immediate appearance of the socket with its prosthesis but also on the future growth of the orbital bones surrounding the socket. The bones of the socket will not grow normally to an adult size if there is nothing inside the socket that enlarges in size and mimics what the natural eye would have done during the childhood growth period. If the bones of the orbit are not stimulated to grow, the appearance of the face can become obviously lopsided. Trying to imitate a growing eye in an infant's socket is not easy to accomplish without multiple surgeries at different times throughout the child's life. A surgeon will try to insert the largest, nonporous implant into the pediatric socket without risking an extrusion of an oversized implant. As the child grows, this implant will be replaced with a larger implant many months or a few years later. This will continue until the child's face reaches a stable size and the sockets appear equal on both sides. Progressively enlarging conformers, which are sutured behind the eyelids, are also used to expand a socket. Pediatric socket expanders are also available; these devices are like thick, hollow balloons that are inserted into the socket. They can be filled with water periodically using a syringe and needle without the need for additional surgery, although the child will need to be put to sleep in a surgery center in order to accomplish this. Dermis-fat grafts inserted into the pediatric orbit have been shown to actually grow and stimulate orbital bone growth.[16]

Whether using progressively enlarging implants, socket expanders, or conformers, the presence of these devices in the socket can stimulate the bones of the orbit to grow simultaneously with the other normal socket. The goal is to create facial symmetry as the infant grows through childhood and into adolescence. If the symmetry is not satisfactory, the child may be sent to a craniofacial surgeon who specializes in expanding the bony orbit with bone grafting and bone expansion techniques.

Pediatric Surgery

When dealing with the socket of an infant or child without an eye, the treatments must begin as soon as possible. Surgeries will often be suggested within the first few weeks or months of life. These surgeries are performed while the infant or child is under general anesthesia. Although no parent ever enjoys knowing that their child requires general anesthesia, the highly sophisticated techniques of pediatric anesthesia have made putting infants and children to sleep for surgery fairly routine at most ambulatory surgery centers and hospitals. Occasionally the very young infant may require a hospital setting that specializes in pediatric surgery and pediatric anesthesia.

Prosthesis

History

Although the actual inventor of the first artificial eye is unknown, there are many accounts throughout history that describe the existence of artificial eyes. A 4,800-year-old artificial eye was found in December 2006 by archaeologist Mansur Sayyed-Sajadis, whose team was working at the Burnt City historical site in southeastern Iran. It is considered to be the world's earliest artificial eyeball, and had a hemispherical shape with a diameter of just over one inch. It was made of a very lightweight material with a tarlike base. The surface of the artificial eye was covered with a thin layer of gold, engraved with a central circle (representing the iris) and gold lines patterned like sun rays. On both sides of the eye were drilled tiny holes, through which a golden thread could hold the eyeball in place. The woman's skeleton has been dated to between 2900 and 2800 BC.[17] The woman with the artificial eye was thought to be between twenty-eight and thirty-two years old. A leather pouch was also found beside the skeleton, which appears to have been used to keep the eye when it was removed.[18]

Ancient artificial eye makers created their works of art more for religious and cosmetic purposes rather than for medical reasons. X-rays of mummies and tombs have discovered artificial eyes made of a variety of materials, such as gold, silver, stones, crystal, shell, and marble. Whereas eye prostheses are fairly common today, their origin is regarded to have come about by accident.

Most of these artificial eyes were worn outside the eyelids, similar to wearing an eye patch. With holes placed on each side, the artistically designed eye was held in place with a string or thread.

Ambrose Pare is credited with the use of artificial eyes made from glass and porcelain.[19] In 1579, the Venetians created what is considered to be the first prosthesis, made of very thin shells of glass that were worn behind the eyelids. The edges were sharp and uncomfortable.

Even William Shakespeare referenced prosthetic eyes in *King Lear*:

> Get three glass eyes;
> And, like a scurvy politician, seem
> To see the things thou dost not.

Advances in prosthetic eyes remained essentially unchanged until 1832, when German glassblower Ludwig Muller-Uri, who made lifelike eyes for dolls, developed a glass eye for his son.

In 1880, Dr. Herman Snellen, inventor of the Snellen vision charting system, developed a thicker, hollow glass prosthesis with rounded edges. His design, called the reform eye design, added significant comfort and wearing time. Germany became the center for producing glass artificial eyes. In 1943, due to the unavailability of glass eyes from Germany during World War II, U.S. Army dental technicians made the first plastic artificial eye. The plastic was difficult to polish on the back side, making them less comfortable than the glass prostheses.

In 1969 Lee Allen, an American artist, ocularist and ophthalmic photographer, developed the modified impression method[20] for producing plastic artificial eyes. This method included a process to duplicate the shape of a patient's socket and modify the front and back surfaces of the prosthesis for comfort. This method is still widely used today.

Ocularist

An ocularist is a skilled medical health professional or technician who is specially trained in the arts of fitting, shaping, designing, and painting ocular prostheses. An ocularist also shows a patient how to take care of their prosthesis.

There are no specific schools or colleges that teach a person to be an ocularist. Ocularists learn how to make artificial eyes by apprenticing with another ocularist and learning the art of creating an ocular prosthesis. Good ocularists are not only technicians but are also artists. Any person who wants to become an ocularist can become one; only a few states in the United States actually regulate this occupation. However, there are two national ocularist organizations that oversee the training and certification of ocularists if they have met certain guidelines and criteria of training.

The American Society of Ocularists (ASO) oversees an apprentice program that requires a student apprentice to study every aspect of ocular prosthesis design and manufacturing. An apprentice must spend five years in practical training with an existing board-approved diplomate ocularist and must successfully complete 750 credits of related study courses offered by the ASO. After successfully completing all requirements, the apprentice is awarded the title of diplomate of the American Society of Ocularists.

Ocularists who pass a comprehensive two-part written and practical examination given by the National Examining Board of Ocularists are then awarded the title of board certified ocularist (BCO). Board certified ocularists must keep on taking continuing education classes throughout their careers in order to become recertified every six years.

Anaplastologist

An anaplastologist is an individual who designs and manufactures facial prostheses. Facial prostheses such as orbital prostheses or maxillofacial prostheses are required to fill in facial defects that are left as a result of surgery to remove large tumors or after severe trauma. It is not uncommon for dentists, dental technicians, or ocularists to become anaplastologists. The anaplastologist will frequently work closely with head and neck surgeons, maxillofacial surgeons, oculoplastic surgeons, and ocularists in developing a prosthesis for a specific region of the face. Typically the anaplastologist will create the prosthesis for a patient who has undergone an exenteration.

There is also a national anaplastologist organization that oversees the training and certification of anaplastologists if they have met certain guidelines and criteria of training. The Board for Certification in Clinical Anaplastology (BCCA) sets the standards for certification by their organization. These standards include strict educational requirements, rigorous certification examinations, mandatory continuing professional education, and professional and ethical guidelines.

Anaplastologists who pass a comprehensive written examination given by the BCCA are then designated as a certified clinical anaplastologist (CCA). Certified clinical anaplastologists must keep taking continuing education classes throughout their careers in order to maintain their certification.

Manufacturing an Ocular Prosthesis

An ocularist making an artificial eye that looks similar to a person's other eye is like an artist painting a picture where the figures look alive. There are a number of manufacturing steps involved in fabricating an ocular prosthesis. Ocular prostheses are made from a medical-grade acrylic called methyl methacrylate.

First, a clear acrylic conformer is placed between the eyelids to open the lids and expose the conjunctival pink wall. An impression of the socket behind the eyelids is then made with an alginate, which is similar to the material that a dentist uses to make a mold of teeth to produce dentures. The impression produces the exact shape, volume, and contour of the socket. A mold is then made of the impression, and a cast is created from the mold with the exact shape as the impression. An acrylic "white blank" is made from the cast.

The details of the eye, which are taken from the existing eye, are then hand painted onto the white blank. The iris or the colored portion of the eye behind the cornea is painted on a flat disc. Matching the color and pattern of this iris disc to the iris of the existing eye is crucial in order to create an equal appearance of the two eyes.

Once the iris is painted, a cornea must be created on top of it. This is produced by layering a clear acrylic over the iris disc until it forms a dome, similar to a cornea. This dome of clear, acrylic material creates a sense of depth in the front part of the eye,

The white blank with the iris and cornea is then fit into the socket to determine comfort, lid shape, and movement. With the white blank placed inside the socket, the iris position is marked. The iris position in relation to the eyelid margins is very important in getting the artificial eye to match the good eye. The completed iris and positioned white blank are then prepared for the final attachment of the iris disc.

Once the iris disc is attached to the white blank, blood vessels (actually red silk threads) are glued to the surface of the white blank to match the other eye. Once the veins are in place, the sclera (white part of the eye) is tinted with acrylic pigments to match the surface patterns and colors of the existing good eye. A final layer of clear acrylic is applied to seal in all of the artwork.

Before the final polishing, adjustments are made to the shape of the prosthesis. Finally, the prosthesis is polished to remove all scratches and produce a surface shine that makes the prosthesis look like a real eye.

From beginning to end, the process of producing a prosthesis typically takes three to four visits with the ocularist spread over one to two weeks. Occasionally, while awaiting the delivery of the final prosthesis, an ocularist may insert a stock prosthesis that has a shape relatively close to the shape of the socket and an iris color close to the patient's existing good eye color.

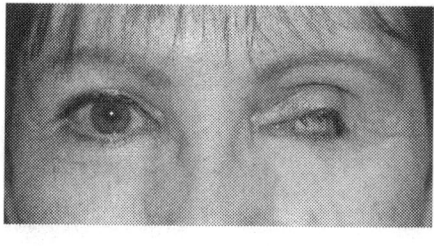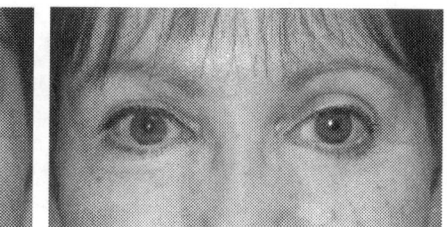

Another material used to make ocular prostheses is silicone (Flexiglass, from Ocular Prosthetic Labs). Making a silicone ocular prosthesis is very similar to producing one in acrylic, however there are a few differences, including the painting and the polishing process. They both take approximately the same amount of time to produce.

Manufacturing an Orbital Prosthesis

An anaplastologist making an orbital prosthesis that looks similar to a person's other orbit and eyelids is like an artist creating a life-like, three-dimensional sculpture. There are a number of manufacturing steps involved in fabricating an orbital prosthesis.

First, an impression is made of both the patient's socket and the normal side using a dental alginate material. Plaster is then poured into the alginate impression to create a model. A wax base plate is then fashioned over the depression in the plaster model, and the artificial eye is inserted. Two more coats of wax are then layered over the wax base plate and the artificial eye. The wax base plate is sculpted to match the character of the other side of the face. This includes eyelids, facial lines, contours, and wrinkles. The space between the eyelids and the height of the eyelids are matched to the other side. The artificial eye is removed from the wax pattern, which is then placed into a denture flask that is used to make dentures. An acrylic material with a predetermined color to match the color of the other side of the face is then packed into the mold. The acrylic is processed and then removed from the flask. The artificial eye is reinserted, and the direction in which the eye is looking is adjusted. If necessary, more sculpting is performed, and occasionally some surface tinting is performed. Eyelashes are attached to the eyelid margins and cemented in place.

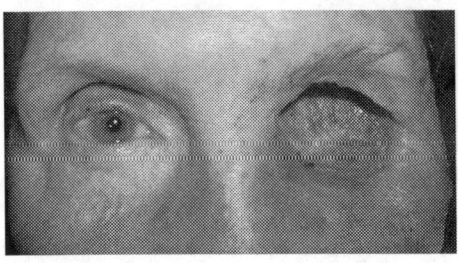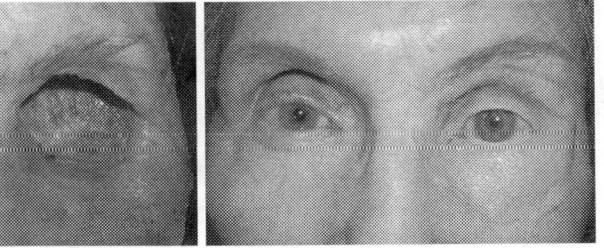

There are a variety of methods that can be used to hold an orbital prosthesis in place. These methods are divided into two categories: implant-retained and adhesive-retained. Skin adhesives can be used to glue the edges of the prosthesis to the skin over the bones of the orbital rim. The prosthesis can be attached to the frame of a pair of glasses as a means of securing the orbital prosthesis against the face and into the open socket. Magnets and pegs (osseointegration) are also used to fasten an orbital prosthesis to the rim of the socket.

From beginning to end, the process of producing an orbital prosthesis typically takes three to four visits with the anaplastologist over one to two weeks.

Care and Handling of an Ocular Prosthesis

For the general health and well-being of the socket, an ocular prosthesis needs to be worn at all times, even while asleep; it should only be removed briefly for cleaning. A bathroom mirror is a good place for removal because a bright light is needed, and the sink provides an area to wash your hands before touching the prosthesis. The sink drain should be closed and the sink covered with a towel to prevent loss of the prosthesis or cracking and scratching if it is accidentally dropped into the sink.

Removal of the prosthetic eye can be done in two different ways. Most people prefer removing it by hand. Both hands must be thoroughly washed with a gentle antibacterial soap. OcuSoft Hand Soap is oil, dye, and fragrance-free so that there's no harmful transfer of oils or lotions (which most soaps contain) from the hands to the prosthesis to the socket. It is also antibacterial and alcohol-free. Other examples of safe soaps to use include Neutrogena, Ivory bar, Opti-Soap, Dial, and any clear dishwashing liquid soap like Joy. After hand washing, it is very important to thoroughly rinse the soap off of the hands before touching the prosthesis. Soap that touches the conjunctival lining of the socket can sting and burn just as badly as getting soap in the good eye.

While looking up, one fingertip is placed over the lower eyelid and used to gently press inward toward the back of the eye socket. This will cause the lower edge of the prosthesis to rotate outward, allowing the other hand to grasp the lower edge and slide the prosthesis out over the lower lid margin. If removing the prosthesis by hand is too difficult, a small, soft rubber suction cup can be used. These suction cups can be obtained directly from an ocularist, online, or sometimes from an ophthalmologist or optometrist. To create the suction with the suction cup, the hollow stem or handle of the suction cup is pinched together, and then the suction cup end is applied to the front of the prosthesis. Releasing the pressure on the stem or handle will allow the suction cup to stick to the prosthesis. The handle can then be rotated upward to release the bottom edge of the prosthesis from the socket and clear the lower lid margin. The handle with the prosthesis still attached is then moved downward to slide the entire prosthesis from under the upper lid. A small amount of white or clear mucous discharge around and behind the prosthesis may be present. These secretions are normal and help the prosthesis feel comfortable while in place.

Cleaning the prosthesis is very important to prevent infection, increase comfort, and also keep it looking realistic and new. Most ocularists recommend removing and cleaning the prosthesis one or two times per week. Alcohol should never be used because it may remove the shine and make the prosthesis appear dull. Abrasives such as toothpaste or denture cleaner should never be used to clean a prosthesis, either. If the prosthesis has a lot of deposits built up on it, it can be soaked in hydrogen peroxide for three to four hours to help loosen the debris; it can then be washed by hand in warm water with a gentle "no tear" soap, such as baby shampoo. The prosthesis should be thoroughly rinsed off before replacing it into the socket, to avoid burning and stinging caused by residual soap.

While the prosthesis is out, the eye socket should also be cleaned using a sterile saline or eye wash solution. This can be squirted into the socket using a syringe or squeeze bottle. An eye cup can also be used to rinse out any secretions. The prosthesis should then be dried with a clean, lint-free towel, and a lubricating solution should be applied to the surface of the prosthesis. It can then be replaced into the socket, either by hand or by using the rubber suction cup.

The insertion process is essentially the reverse of the removal process. The prosthesis is typically inserted under the upper eyelid first and then pushed back to clear the lower eyelid margin. Once past the lower eyelid margin, the prosthesis can then be pushed up, over, and behind the lower lid margin and released. Occasionally, a slight downward pull on the lower eyelid will assure that the lower edge of the prosthesis will fall behind the lower lid margin. Most people will insert the prosthesis by hand even if they remove it with a suction cup. If the suction cup is used to insert it, then squeezing the stem or handle with the thumb and forefinger will release the suction when the prosthesis has cleared the lower lid margin.

Polishing and cleaning should be done professionally by the ocularist at least once or twice per year. This provides a deeper cleaning and removes any buildup of minerals, debris, protein deposits, or bacteria. It will also extend the life of the prosthesis and ensure that it looks its best. The ocularist will also closely inspect the prosthesis to look for small cracks or rough areas that may need to be polished or smoothed over. Protein deposits and some secretions can lodge themselves inside small cracks and scratches which allow more protein to build up. Each cleaning and polishing with the local ocularist should take less than an hour and can save money in the long run by increasing the longevity of the prosthesis.

Ocular prostheses typically need to be replaced about every four to five years. If the tissues of the socket surrounding the prosthesis change, then this can lead to an undesirable fit or discomfort, and the prosthesis may have to be modified sooner. Also, irreparable scratches or damage may require complete replacement of the prosthesis altogether. The older prostheses that were made of glass wore out quicker and broke very easily. Today, plastic is the material of choice due to its durability and strength. Though glass prostheses usually need to be replaced every year or two, people who wear plastic prostheses can often go up to five to seven years or even longer if the prostheses are well taken care of.

Warning signs of a possible infection include excessive discharge or tearing, a change in discharge (from white or clear to green or yellow color), redness or swelling of the tissues surrounding the prosthesis, excessive itching, and unusual pain or discomfort. If any of these signs or symptoms develops, an eye doctor should be consulted to remove the prosthesis and thoroughly examine the socket. If a cold or sinus infection is present, the amount of secretions may increase and change consistency or color; this can also occur with seasonal allergies.

Lubricating the prosthesis frequently is the best way to ensure that the eyelids do not stick to the surface. It also allows the prosthesis to move easier, appear realistic, and feel more comfortable.

There are basically three types of ocular lubricants: water-based ophthalmic drops and gels, petrolatum-based ophthalmic ointments, and silicone-based oil drops. One of the best methods to keep a prosthesis well lubricated is to use an over-the-counter artificial tear ointment three to four times per day. Artificial teardrops may also be used, but these tend to evaporate very quickly, providing only about fifteen minutes of relief. Enuclene (from Alcon Laboratories) contains tyloxapol and is used in cleaning, lubricating, and wetting artificial eyes. Tyloxapol is a liquid drop used to melt away mucopurulent (containing mucus and pus) and protein deposits from the surface of an ocular prosthesis. Tears Again Liquid Gel Drops (from Cynacon/Ocusoft) is a popular product among ocular prosthesis wearers. Its viscosity is thicker than artificial tear drops but thinner than artificial tear ointments.

Ophthalmic ointments, on the other hand, contain petrolatum, mineral oil, and sometimes lanolin, which stay on the surface of the prosthesis for hours. Some examples of ophthalmic ointments include Lacrilube, Refresh PM, Tears Natural PM, Genteal PM, Puralube, and Advanced Eye Relief Night Time. Gently pulling the lower lid down will provide an area to squeeze about one-quarter to one-half inch of ointment just below the prosthesis.

There is a definite difference between lubricant and moisturizers for normal eyes and lubricants exclusively made for artificial eyes. The main difference between these two types of lubricants is thickness or viscosity. Normal eye lubricants, commonly called artificial tears, are very thin like water, whereas artificial eye lubricants are much heavier and thicker like vegetable oil. Artificial eye lubricants typically contain silicone, which never really dries completely, unlike artificial tears, which are water based and can dry up or evaporate quickly.

Ocu-Glide (from Doctors Associates Rx Inc.) is a medical-grade, silicone-based prosthetic eye gel specifically designed as an ocular prosthesis lubricant. Ocu-Glide is water resistant, is not absorbed by the body, and provides long lasting results. Ocu-Sil (from MSM Industries, LLC) is a liquid silicone oil used as a lubricant for ocular prostheses. Medical-grade, silicone-based lubricants are frequently recommended by eye doctors and ocularists to improve prosthetic eye comfort, appearance, and movement. Sil-Ophtho and Sil-Ophtho-H (from Stony Brook Inc.) are medium and heavy viscosity silicone-based lubricants, respectively, that are specifically designed for ocular prostheses. Artificial Eye Lubricant (from Strauss Eye Prosthetics, Inc.) is a non-silicone, Vitamin E and Aloe Vera-based lubricant made specifically for artificial eyes.

Kevin V. Kelley, a board-certified ocularist from Philadelphia, Pennsylvania, developed a self-lubricating prosthesis (SLP). The design of the SLP is a typical solid prosthetic eye with an attached flexible chamber above it to store lubricants. The chamber fits below the upper eyelid within the socket and slowly releases lubricants over the front of the prosthesis. This allows for continual surface wetting and improved comfort. The chamber may be easily refilled with the prosthesis in place, simply by removing the cap.

Care and Handling of an Orbital Prosthesis

Unlike an ocular prosthesis, an orbital prosthesis does not need to be worn at all times. If an orbital prosthesis is not worn during the day, an eye patch can be worn over the empty socket to prevent people from looking at the socket. When the orbital prosthesis is worn during the day, it must be removed and left out at night before sleep to allow the surrounding skin a chance to recover from the constant contact with the prosthesis.

Prior to applying the skin adhesive to the skin of the orbital rim, the adhesive-retained prosthesis should be inserted and removed a few times to make sure that its position is accurate. Both hands and the surrounding skin of the orbital rim must be thoroughly washed with a gentle antibacterial soap and completely dried with a clean, lint-free towel.

If adhesive is used, a thin layer of adhesive is spread along the outer edges of the back side of the prosthesis using the brush that comes with the bottle. A cotton-tipped applicator can also be used. The adhesive is not applied to the skin. The adhesive should be allowed to dry until sticky. After positioning the prosthesis, insert it into the socket and press it onto the skin.

When removing an orbital prosthesis, it can be helpful if the surface of the prosthesis near the outer edges is moistened with a wet cloth. This can loosen some of the adhesive. The prosthesis is grabbed at its thickest edge and gently pulled away from the skin. Pulling the prosthesis slowly will help prevent tearing the edges of the prosthesis. The adhesive can be removed off the prosthesis by rolling it off the back surface, starting from the center of the prosthesis and moving toward its outer edge. This will prevent tearing the edge of the prosthesis. This technique can be accomplished with a fingertip, a gauze pad, or a textured cloth.

Smooth cloths do not create enough friction to remove the adhesive. After removal, the prosthesis can be soaked in warm water to soften any residual adhesive and make it easier to remove completely.

If the orbital prosthesis has an ocular prosthesis (artificial eye) as a part of it, the artificial eye should be removed and cleaned separately (see: Prosthesis: Care and Handling of an Ocular Prosthesis). The orbital prosthesis can then be cleaned using a soft, nylon toothbrush and a mild antibacterial soap with warm water. The prosthesis should be stored dry overnight. The artificial eye should be replaced after the orbital prosthesis is completely dry.

Any residual adhesive found on the skin should be thoroughly removed with soap and warm water. Some patients find it helpful to apply a skin moisturizer before bedtime to prevent the skin from becoming dry. Any skin redness or irritation should be reported to the eye doctor immediately. The adhesive should not be applied over irritated skin, and the prosthesis may have to be left out for a few days until the skin returns to normal.

Implant-retained prostheses are mechanically held in the socket using magnets or pegs. Some patients will also apply a small amount of adhesive to the outer edges of these prostheses to keep the prosthesis edges firmly against the skin.

Unlike an ocular prosthesis, an orbital prosthesis will only last about a year and will require a replacement. The time to replace an orbital prosthesis is dependent on surface color change, poor retention in the socket, or tears along the outer edge of the prosthesis.

Life with a Prosthesis

Physical Limitations

Depending on the amount and quality of vision in the remaining eye, a patient may have virtually no physical limitations following removal of an eye. They may still be able to read, watch TV, drive, and easily do other activities that they enjoyed before surgery. However, two eyes are required for the perception of depth. It takes time to get used to life with one eye when it comes to certain tasks. For example, placing toothpaste on a toothbrush may prove a bit more challenging at first. Pouring coffee into a cup may result in spills. Sewing or crocheting may be difficult. Caution must be taken especially when walking up or down stairs, or stepping off a curb into a street. Driving and parking a car may be difficult for quite some time. In some cases, a person with only one eye may not feel comfortable enough driving at all. A person who has recently lost an eye may find it very helpful to practice pulling into many of the marked parking spaces in an empty shopping mall parking lot when no other cars are around. This exercise can help reestablish a sense of depth perception while driving. Initially, someone else should be in the car to assist until a certain level of comfort is reached. Special extra-long rearview mirrors can be very helpful in compensating for the reduced side vision on the side of the lost eye.

Occupational Hazards

Unfortunately, certain occupations are not compatible with having one eye. Some occupations require a wide range of peripheral vision to avoid potentially dangerous situations. For example, police officers, airline pilots, commercial truck drivers, and firefighters are required to have excellent vision in both eyes. Other occupations rely heavily on good depth perception to accomplish the duties associated with the job—surgeons, architects, crane and forklift operators, high altitude construction workers, and some athletes. For a construction worker with one eye, operating a table saw or hammering a nail could be difficult and potentially hazardous at first. For a seamstress, threading a needle can be extremely frustrating. For a chef, liquids poured into a bowl or pan may end up on the floor or in the flames of the cooking top. The waitress may miss the glass and pour the water on the table or in the lap of the customer. The salesman may not immediately notice a customer standing to the side of his or her prosthesis until a slight head turn is made.

Fortunately, most occupations are completely unaffected by having one eye. Even more fortunate is that after a brief relearning period, the vast majority of these tasks can be compensated for and easily accomplished without any problems. However, it does require some time and effort to retrain the brain to get used to functioning with only one eye after a lifetime with two.

A job-related loss of an eye qualifies a worker as having lost 25 percent of his or her visual system and 24 percent of the total body system. Workman's compensation agencies that deal with work-related eye injuries utilize these standardized figures to compute compensation.

Protecting the Good Eye

Anyone who has poor or absent vision in one eye must take extra precautions to protect the good or better eye. Special protective glasses made of very strong polycarbonate material should be worn at all times. The purpose of these glasses is to prevent anything from causing loss of vision in the only remaining eye. Even if the injury (for example, a corneal abrasion) only requires patching the injured eye for twenty-four hours, that represents a day of total blindness in the patient with a prosthesis. Prescription glasses can be made out of this shatterproof material, if desired; traditional eye glasses, made of glass or plastic, can break very easily and should not be worn. Polycarbonate is a very thin, lightweight material that also happens to block the harmful ultraviolet rays from the sun. In fact, this material is so strong that children's glasses, sport goggles, and safety goggles are also made of polycarbonate. Bulletproof glass is made of this as well. Glasses made of this material may be slightly more expensive but are well worth the protective benefits.

The quality and durability of the frame of the glasses is just as important as the lenses in the glasses. The frame of the glasses must also be able to withstand an accidental impact without collapsing or breaking, which could cause further injury to the good eye. Flimsy or delicate wire frames do not offer as much protection as frames made of the same polycarbonate materials as the lenses.

Additional protection is absolutely necessary when performing any activity where a foreign body could potentially be projected toward the good eye. This means wearing a pair of safety glasses on top of the protective glasses or in place of the protective glasses. If the protective glasses have a prescription in the lens for the good eye, then the safety glasses should be worn over the prescription glasses. The safety glasses should be of the goggle type to prevent anything from flying into the eye from the side.

Swimming should be done only with goggles on to protect the good eye from irritation from the water, if chemically treated, or from a potential infection caused by microorganisms in untreated water such as lakes or ponds. Goggles will also prevent the loss of the prosthesis if it should accidentally fall out while swimming.

In addition, anyone who has poor or absent vision in one eye needs to have more frequent eye examinations. This means visiting their eye doctor at least once a year to have the good eye fully examined. The doctor will check vision and eye pressure and may dilate the eye to examine the inside of the eye as well. Some patients may need a visual field test done by a machine to document their range of side vision for purposes of driving.

Most surgeons will be somewhat reluctant to perform any surgery on the only eye of a one-eyed person unless it is absolutely medically necessary. The benefits of that surgery must totally outweigh the risks of surgery. Because the majority of eye surgeries carry a risk of blindness to that eye, careful considerations must be made before proceeding with any surgery on the only eye.

In a world where the overwhelming majority of people have two eyes, the absence of one eye certainly does not reduce the quality of life by half. In fact, it minimally reduces the quality of what is seen. Viewing the world through one good eye captures the same images as the single lens of a camera captures them in photographs. With today's surgical advances in eyelid and orbital reconstruction, and with the technical advances in manufacturing and fabricating eye and orbital prostheses, the only person who may recognize that an individual is missing an eye is the person himself.

Glossary of Terminology

acrylic	A material made of plastic.
adhesive-retained	A method of holding an orbital prosthesis in the socket using glue placed on the skin.
alginate	A material extensively used in dentistry to make impressions of the mouth and teeth.
amniotic membrane	The outer layer of the birth sac that contains the fetus.
analgesics	Drugs that are used to reduce pain.
anaplastologist	A person who designs and manufactures orbital and facial prostheses.
anophthalmos	A socket that does not contain a natural eye.

antibiotic	Medicine used to kill bacteria causing an infection.
aqueous	Clear fluid produced by the ciliary body that fills the front portion of the inside of the eye.
bilateral	Both sides or both eyes.
biopsy	The sample of tissue removed by surgery that is evaluated by a pathologist to determine the exact kind of tissue.
cataract	The natural crystalline lens of the eye that has become cloudy or opaque as a result of aging or disease.
Charles Bonnet syndrome	A disease that causes patients with visual loss to have visual hallucinations.
chemosis	A severe swelling of the conjunctiva.
chemotherapy	Using drugs and other medications to treat patients with cancer.
choroid	A layer of the eye between the sclera and retina that contains a lot of blood vessels, which nourish both of these layers.

ciliary body	A part of the inside of the eye that produces the fluid that fills the inside of the eye.
conformer	A half-almond, shell-shaped, clear piece of plastic used to keep the curved shape of the eyelids.
congenital	Condition with which a person is born.
conjunctiva	A clear mucous membrane that covers the white sclera and the inside of the eyelids.
conjunctivitis	An inflammation or infection of the conjunctiva.
cornea	The clear "window" in the front of the eye where light enters.
craniofacial surgeon	A surgeon who specializes in surgery involving the bones of the skull and face.
denture flask	A container used in the production of dentures.
dermis	One of the many layers of the skin that lies just below the surface.
dermis-fat graft	A composite graft consisting of both the dermis and fat.

donor site	A location from where a graft (e.g., skin) comes.
ectropion	An abnormal position of the lower eyelid where the eyelid turns away from the eyeball or prosthesis.
endophthalmitis	A severe infection involving the inside of the eye which can cause blindness.
enophthalmos	An abnormal position of the eyeball where the eye sinks back into the socket.
entropion	An abnormal position of the eyelid where the eyelid turns in toward from the eyeball or prosthesis.
enucleation	Surgery that removes the entire eyeball.
evisceration	Surgery that only removes the inner contents of the eyeball and leaves the outer shell (ie, the scleral) intact.
exenteration	Surgery that removes all or part of the structures of the orbit that includes the eyelids, eyeball, eye muscles and orbital fat.
extraocular muscle	Muscles that are attached to the outside of the eye which are responsible for eye movements.

extrusion	Forced out of the socket (pertaining to an orbital implant).
fascia	Soft tissue that surrounds and connects different body parts with each other.
fornix (plural: fornices)	The grooves in the upper and lower conjunctiva where the conjunctiva that covers the scleral meets the conjunctiva that covers the inside of the eyelids.
giant papillary conjunctivitis	A condition of the conjunctiva that covers the inside of the upper eyelid characterized by small elevations or bumps (i.e., papillae) that produce mucous.
glaucoma	A condition of the eye characterized by a high pressure inside the eye which damages the optic nerve and reduces peripheral (side) vision and can lead to blindness, if untreated.
goblet cells	Specialized cells of the conjunctiva that produce mucous for the tear film.
granuloma	Small growth of conjunctiva near an area of irritation.
hemorrhage	Excessive bleeding inside or outside the body.

immune system	A collection of biological processes in the body that protects against disease and infection.
implant-retained	A method of holding an orbital prosthesis in the socket using magnets or pegs.
incompetent socket	A socket that will not hold a prosthesis in place.
infection	Harmful effect of microorganisms (eg, bacteria) in or on a body tissue.
inflammation	A biological response of the body tissue to something harmful.
integrateable implant	A volume-occupying object inserted into the eye socket to replace the eye which can later be attached to the prosthesis.
iris	Colored portion of the eye.
lacrimal	Pertaining to the parts of the orbit responsible for producing and drainage of tears.
lacrimal gland	Soft tissue structure that produces tears located in the upper outer corner of the orbit.

lens	Clear structure in the eye that focuses light onto the retina.
meibomian gland	Small structures located in the eyelids that produce oil.
malignant	Referring to cancers that have a tendency to spread and eventually cause death.
microorganisms	Living structures that can cause infection such as bacteria, viruses and fungi.
monocular	Having one eye.
motility peg	A small metal or plastic device attached to the orbital implant that sticks out of the socket to integrate with the prosthesis for better movement.
moulage	A molded impression of the socket that contains the eyelids and an artificial eye.
mucopurulent	A discharge containing a mixture of mucous and pus.
mucous membrane	A layer of cells that covers the inside of the mouth, nose and sinuses and produces mucous to stay moist.
necrosis	Destruction of body tissue.

nonporous implant	A solid, spherical, marble-shaped ball used to replace the orbital volume left when an eye is removed.
ocularist	A person who designs and manufactures artificial eyes and prostheses.
occipital lobe	The portion of the brain in the back of the skull responsible for vision.
open globe	An eyeball that has been cut open as a result of an injury.
optic nerve	An extension of the brain into the back of the eyeball that transmits visual signals from the retina to the brain.
orbit	The cavity surrounded by bones where the eyeball is located; the socket.
orbital implant	A volume-occupying object inserted into the eye socket to replace the eye.
osseointegration	A method of holding an orbital prosthesis in place using metal pegs that are inserted into the bones of the orbit. The prosthesis clips onto the pegs.
papillae	Elevated bumps of conjunctival tissue found on the inside of the eyelids.

phthisical eye	An eye with no internal pressure that usually shrinks into a small, collapsed shape.
polycarbonate	A plastic material that can be made shatterproof and unbreakable. It is used in producing safety glasses.
porous implant	A spherical, marble-shaped ball filled with tiny holes and channels used to replace the orbital volume left when an eye is removed.
prosthesis (plural: prostheses)	Artificial replacement part (e.g., artificial eye).
prosthetic stare	A wide open eye appearance that makes the prosthesis appear to be gazing directly at someone or something.
ptosis	Drooping upper eyelids.
pupil	A circular hole in the center of the iris that regulates the amount of light that enters the back of the eye.
radiation therapy	Treatment using high beam X-rays to control and destroy cancer cells.
rectus muscles	Eye muscles that move the eye up, down, right, and left.

retina	The transparent inner layer of the back of the eye that receives light and transmits the visual signals to the brain.
sclera	The white outer layer of the eyeball.
silicone	A chemical compound used as a lubricant that does not dissolve in water and spreads very well over most surfaces.
socket	The cavity surrounded by bones where the eyeball is located; the orbit.
steroid	Medicine used to reduce inflammation.
superior sulcus deformity	A depression or hollowness found in the upper eyelid just below the eyebrow caused by a loss of orbital volume.
symblepharon	Scarring of the conjunctiva.
sympathetic ophthalmia	A condition where the uninjured good eye "sympathizes" with the injured eye and can develop a significant inflammatory response, which can lead to reduced vision and even blindness.

vascularization	Growth of blood vessels into a tissue of the body or into an implant (e.g., porous implant).
viscosity	The thickness or stickiness of a liquid.
vitreous	A clear, gel-like liquid that fills the back portion of the inside of the eye.
wound dehiscence	The separation of the edges of a recently stitched surgical wound.

Endnotes

1 Hansen AB, Peterson C, Heegaard S, Prause JU. Review of 1028 bulbar eviscerations and enucleations. Changes in aetiology and frequency over a 20-year period. Acta Ophthalmol Scand. 1999; 77(3): 331–5.

2 www.weironline.org/prevention.htm.

3 Smith D, Wrenn K, Stack LB. The epidemiology and diagnosis of penetrating eye injuries. Acad Emerg Med. 2002; 9(3): 209–213.

4 http://www.aao.org/newsroom/guide/upload/Eye-Injuries-BkgrnderLongVersFinal-l.pdf.

5 Koval R, et al. The Israeli Ocular Injuries Study: A Nationwide Collaborative Study. Arch Ophthalmol. 1988; 106(6): 776–780.

6 Negrel AD, Thylefors B. The global impact of eye injuries. Ophthalmic Epidemiol. 1998; 5(3): 143–69.

7 United States Eye Injury Registry. http://www.useironline.org.

8 Maguire P, Parkes CM. Coping with loss: Surgery and loss of body parts. *BMJ.* 1998; 316: 1086–1088

9 http://www.eyecancer.com/Patient/Treatment.aspx?nID=2&Treatment=Enucleation+Surgery+-+Removal+of+the+Eye.

10 Menon GJ, Rahman I, Menon SJ, Dutton GN.. Complex visual hallucinations in the visually impaired: The Charles Bonnet Syndrome. Surv Ophthalmol. 2003 Jan–Feb; 48(1): 58–72

11 http://artificialretina.energy.gov. Last modified: February 27, 2008.

12 Marak GE. Recent advances in sympathetic ophthalmia. Surv Ophthalmol. 1979;24: 141–146.

13 Rubin JR, Albert DM, Weinstein M. Sixty-five years of sympathetic ophthalmia: a clinical review of 105 cases (1913-1978). Ophthalmol. 1980; 87: 109–121.

14 Bartisch G. Ophthalmodoulica oder Augendienst, Dresden, 1583.

15 Luce CM. A short history of enucleation. Int Ophthalmol Clin. 1970; 10: 681–687.

16 Heher KL, Katowitz JA, Low JE. Unilateral dermis-fat graft implantation in the pediatric orbit. Ophthal Plast Reconstr Surg. 1998 Mar; 14(2): 81–8.

17 Ancient Artificial Eye Unearthed in Iran. Jennifer Viegas, Discovery News, Dec. 18, 2006.

18 The Circle of Ancient Iranian Studies News, Mar 9, 2009.

19 Soll DB: Evolution and Current concepts in the Treatment of the Anophthalmic Orbit. In Smith BC, Della Rocca RC, Nesi FA, Lisman RD, editors:Ophthalmic Plastic and Reconstructive Surgery, St. Louis, Missouri,1987, CV Mosby Company.

20 Allen L, Webster HE. Modified impression method of artificial eye fitting. Am J Ophthalmol 1969; 67: 189.